SURGICAL CRITICAL CARE

Robert U. Ashford, MBBS, MRCS(Glasg)
Specialist Registrar in
Trauma & Orthopaedic Surgery
South Trent Deanery
UK

T Neal Evans, MBBS, FRCA
Specialist Registrar in Anaesthesia
Oxford Deanery
UK

GMM
LONDON SAN FRANCISCO

G M M

© 2001

Greenwich Medical Media Limited.
137 Euston Road
London
NW1 2AA

870 Market Street, Ste 720
San Francisco CA 94109, USA

ISBN 1 84110 0668

First Published 2001

www.greenwich-medical.co.uk

Distributed worldwide by Plymbridge Distributors Ltd

Typeset by Saxon Graphics Limited, Derby

Printed in Great Britain by Alden Press Ltd, UK

CONTENTS

PREFACE

Critical care plays an increased role in surgical practice. Most junior surgical doctors care for numerous patients who require intensive care or high dependency support. The Royal Colleges have recognised the importance of critical care, incorporating it into the new MRCS examination as a viva section specifically, and in three sections of the MCQ papers (ITU, preoperative and postoperative management). Obviously, it also plays a part in all the other subsections. Critical care also features prominently in the intercollegiate FRCS (Gen) examination.

The contents of this book have been based on the MRCS syllabus of the Royal College of Surgeons of England. Whilst the book is principally aimed as a revision guide for those undertaking the MRCS examination, it will also be useful to those working on a surgical ITU. We hope those of you using this book as a revision guide will be successful in the examination. To facilitate revision, the book has been extensively cross-referenced to both *Clinical Surgery in General* (The Royal College of Surgeons of England, 3rd edition) and *Surgery* (The Medicine Publishing Group).

We are indebted to those who have made this book possible. Andrew Archbold deserves special tribute for his very significant contribution to the cardiovascular section. The contributions of Tim Jones and Richard Downs are also much appreciated. Kumar Panikkar and Robert McCarthy have undertaken the task of proof reading enthusiastically and to them we offer our gratitude. The knowledge and helpful advice of Gavin Smith, Geoff Nuttall, Nora Naughton and her team is also appreciated. Finally, our sincere thanks to our wives, Isabel and Annabelle for their support, encouragement and understanding during the preparation of the book.

Rob Ashford
Neal Evans
Sheffield & Oxford 2001

FOREWORD

Junior Surgeons are often in the front line in the management of the critically ill patient. At such times knowledge and practical skills that have been learned and properly understood, are essential. This text provides an extensive, easily read, easily memorable yet concise narrative of the pathophysiology, management and treatment of these conditions.

The reader will find a wealth of knowledge woven into the flow diagrams, algorithms and bullet-point lists that reinforce the factual text material and serve as excellent aide mémoire for examinations.

The authors are to be particularly commended on their frequent cross-referencing to further reading: in particular to the excellent series of articles written in the journal "Surgery" from the Medicine Publishing Company.

Besides the theoretic knowledge, the authors have provided a very useful section on Practical Procedures, which outlines the essential step-by-step techniques involved. Robert Ashford and Neal Evans have assembled a highly readable text that will become a leading text in the field of critical care in surgery.

Andrew N. Kingsnorth BSc MS FRCS FACS
Professor of Surgery
University of Plymouth, UK
Member, Court of Examiners
Royal College of Surgeons of England

CONTRIBUTORS

R. Andrew Archbold MB, BS (Lond.), MRCP (UK)
Specialist Registrar in Cardiology
North Thames Deanery (East)
UK

Robert U. Ashford, MB, BS (Lond.), MRCS (Glasg)
Specialist Registrar in Trauma & Orthopaedic Surgery
South Trent Deanery
UK

Richard Downs MB, BS (Lond.) FRCA
Consultant in Anaesthesia and Intensive Care
Stoke Mandeville Hospital
Aylesbury
UK

T. Neal Evans, MBBS (Lond.), FRCA
Specialist Registrar in Anaesthetics
Oxford Deanery
UK

Timothy J. Jones, MB, BS (Lond.) FRCS
Specialist Registrar in Cardiothoracic Surgery
West Midlands Deanery
UK

Robert J. McCarthy, MB BS (Lond.) FRCS
Specialist Registrar in General Surgery
South West Deanery
UK

Kumar Panikkar, MBBS (Lond.) FRCA
Director of Intensive Care
Stoke Mandeville Hospital
Aylesbury
UK

1

CARDIOVASCULAR

Cardiac Output: Physiology and Pharmacology

Cardiac Arrest and Resuscitation

Clinical Assessment and Invasive Monitoring of Volume Status, Cardiac Output and Systemic Vascular Resistance

Electrocardiography and Echocardiography in the Surgical Patient

Management of Haemorrhage and Shock

Pulmonary Oedema

General Principles of Cardiopulmonary Bypass

Haematological Problems

Postoperative Complications of Cardiothoracic Surgery

CARDIAC OUTPUT: PHYSIOLOGY AND PHARMACOLOGY

R. Andrew Archbold

Physiology of cardiac output

Cardiac output is the volume of blood ejected from the left ventricle per minute

Cardiac output = stroke volume × heart rate

$$CO = SV \times HR.$$

Stroke volume and hence cardiac output, is dependent on filling pressure (pre-load), the resistance imparted by the systemic circulation (afterload) and myocardial contractility.

Starling's Law

The force of myocardial muscle contraction is proportional to the amount of stretch in the cardiac muscle fibres before contraction. Thus, in the normal heart, stroke volume increases as the end-diastolic volume increases (Starling's Law) (Figure 1.1).

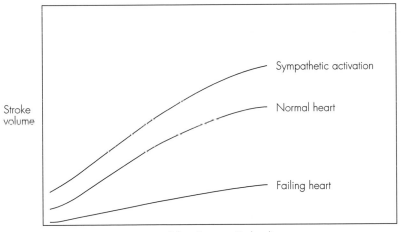

Figure 1.1: Ventricular function curves demonstrating the relationship between stroke volume and preload in the normal, failing and stimulated heart.

Table 1.1: Displacement of ventricular function curve.

Upward displacement (increased contractility)	Downward displacement (decreased contractility)
Sympathetic activation Positive inotropes	Hypoxia Acidosis Negative inotropes (β-blockers, calcium antagonists)

The ventricular function curve is displaced as indicated in Table 1.1.

Myocardial contractility and stroke volume are also related to afterload such that a decrease in peripheral vascular resistance at a given preload results in an increase in stroke volume. High afterload also increases myocardial work and oxygen demands.

Pathophysiology of heart failure

As the heart begins to fail, physiological changes occur which seek to correct the inability of the heart to maintain cardiac output at normal filling pressures.

- The reduction in stroke volume is accompanied by an increase in end-diastolic volume.

- The resulting increase in myocardial muscle stretching promotes improved contractility with restoration of stroke volume.

- Reduced renal blood flow activates the renin—angiotensin—aldosterone system causing sodium and water retention, which contribute to the increase in preload. Angiotensin also causes vasoconstriction, which helps to maintain systemic blood pressure.

- The sympathetic nervous system is activated resulting in an increase in heart rate that compensates for the reduction in stroke volume (CO = SV × HR), and an increase in myocardial contractility through stimulation of β_1-adrenoceptors.

In the failing heart, however, the left ventricular function curve is flattened (Figure 1.1) such that increasing left atrial filling pressures (> 20 mmHg) do not produce an increase in stroke volume, but do predispose to the development of pulmonary venous hypertension and pulmonary oedema.

Atrial fibrillation and cardiac output

In sinus rhythm, blood flows passively from the atria into the ventricles in early diastole before atrial contraction in late diastole augments ventricular filling. In atrial fibrillation (AF), effective mechanical atrial contraction is lost and a decrease in cardiac output of up to 25% may result (Table 1.2).

Table 1.2: Mechanisms contributing to the adverse haemodynamic consequences of AF.

Loss of atrial contraction
Tachycardia (reduced diastolic filling and coronary perfusion time)
Irregular ventricular contraction
Atrioventricular (mitral and tricuspid) valve regurgitation

Optimisation of cardiac output

Cardiac output can be influenced favourably by the optimisation of preload, after-load and myocardial contractility. Mechanical circulatory support and control of arrhythmias may also be appropriate.

Optimisation of preload

Volume status can be assessed both clinically and by invasive monitoring such as central venous and pulmonary artery flotation catheterisation (see Clinical assessment and invasive monitoring of volume status, cardiac output and systemic vascular resistance, and Chapter 6, Pulmonary Artery Flotation Catheter).

Initial resuscitation in the hypotensive patient typically involves Hartmann's solution for trauma and colloids in other circumstances. Thereafter, the **hypovolaemic patient** should be resuscitated with fluids that reflect the fluid compartment from which the volume has been lost (Table 1.3).

Table 1.3: Appropriate replacement of fluid loss

Scenario	Fluid replacement
Acute blood loss	Cross-matched blood (available within 1 h) or type specific (15 min)
Catastrophic haemorrhage	Group O Rhesus-negative blood (immediate)
Extracellular fluid losses (e.g. vomiting, diarrhoea and intra-abdominal losses)	saline supplemented by potassium
Septic shock	Volume replacement (colloid and crystalloid) to compensate for vasodilatation and fluid leakage resulting from loss of the integrity of the capillary bed

In spontaneously breathing patients a right-sided filling pressure (CVP) of 10–12 mmHg and a left-sided filling pressure (PAOP) of 16–18 mmHg usually indicates an appropriate preload to optimise cardiac output. Occasionally volume replacement to achieve higher right-sided filling pressures are warranted, e.g. right ventricular infarction, pulmonary embolism, cardiac tamponade.

In the **volume-overloaded patient**, the preload/filling pressures are elevated and should be reduced with venodilators, e.g. IV glyceryl trinitrate and diuresis with IV furosemide (frusemide). The flat ventricular function curve in the failing heart means that the stroke volume is not decreased further by the reduction in preload. The pulmonary venous pressure, however, is reduced below the threshold for the development of pulmonary oedema (20–25 mmHg), improving oxygenation.

Afterload

Afterload reduction may improve stroke volume and reduce myocardial oxygen demands, particularly in the hypertensive patient. Vasodilators such as sodium nitroprusside and hydralazine can be used as IV infusions and titrated according to the response.

Control of systemic blood pressure is especially important in the management of aortic dissection. This applies equally to type A dissections (which involve the ascending aorta) before definitive surgery and type B dissections (which do not involve the ascending aorta), the management of which is medical. In this setting, infusions of sodium nitroprusside and labetalol are frequently used to lower blood pressure.

Vasoactive agents

Several different positive inotropes exist which can be used in an attempt to increase the contractility of the heart (Table 1.4).

Dopamine

The effects of dopamine are related to the dosage:

- Low-dose ($< 5 \ \mu g \ kg^{-1} min^{-1}$) dopamine dilates renal, cerebral, coronary and splanchnic vessels through stimulation of pre- (D1) and post- (D2) synaptic dopaminergic receptors and β_1-adrenoceptors resulting in increased cardiac contractility and heart rate.

- High-dose ($> 10 \ \mu g \ kg^{-1} min^{-1}$) dopamine stimulates α-adrenoceptors causing vasoconstriction.

Dobutamine

Dobutamine is termed an inodilator and stimulates β_1- and β_2-adrenoceptors in the heart (increasing myocardial contractility) and peripherally (mediating vasodilatation). It is less likely to cause tachycardia or peripheral vasoconstriction than dopamine and is generally regarded as the inotrope of first choice in the management of cardiogenic shock due to left ventricular dysfunction.

Clinically, dobutamine and low-dose dopamine are frequently used together in the management of cardiogenic shock in an attempt to increase blood pressure

Table 1.4: Vasoactive agents used to manipulate the circulation.

Drug	Presentation	Concentration for infusion (in 50 mls dextrose)	Infusion rate (µg/kg⁻ min)	Effects on:				Mechanism of action	Indications
				HR	CO	BP	SVR		
Adrenaline (epinephrine)	5 mg in 5 mls	100 µg/ml	0.1–0.25	↑	↑	↑	↑↓ / ↑	mainly β α with ↑ dose	Cardiac failure – to incrase inotropic function
Noradrenaline (norepinephrine)	4 mg in 5 mls	80 µg/ml	0.02–0.4	→↓	↑→↓	↑	↑↑	mainly α	Sepsis
Dopamine	200 mg in 5 mls	4 mg ml⁻¹	3–5 >10	↑↑ ↑↑	↑↑ ↑↓	→↑ ↑	→↓ / ↑	DA + β mainly α	↑ Volume of urine output in acute renal failure
Dobutamine	250 mg in 5 mls	5 mg ml⁻¹	2–20	↑	↑	→↑	→	β₁ β₂	Cardiac failure – to decrease afterload
Dopexamine	50 mg in 5 mls	1 mg ml⁻¹	0.5–6	↑	↑	→↑	→	β₂	Cardiac failure – to decrease afterload and improve splanchnic perfusion
Isoprenaline	4 mg in 5 mls	80 µg/ml	0.05–0.8	↑↑	↑	→↑	→↓	β₁	Chronotype – used for heart block (until paced)
GTN	50 mg in 50 mls	1 mg ml⁻¹	0.2–3	→↑	→↓	→	→	Production of NO	Cardiac failure – to decrease preload

(through increased cardiac contractility) and urine output (through increased renal perfusion) respectively.

Dopexamine

Dopexamine acts primarily on β_2-adrenoceptors and dopaminergic (DA) receptors. This results in inotropic and chronotropic action (especially in the failing heart), increased peripheral vasodilatation, increased splanchnic blood flow and increased renal perfusion leading to improved urine output (diuresis).

Adrenaline (epinephrine)

Adrenaline stimulates both α- and β-adrenoceptors. At low doses a β-mediated increase in cardiac contractility predominates, while at higher doses α-mediated vasoconstriction occurs. This can increase peripheral vascular resistance (afterload) and myocardial oxygen demands with an adverse effect on cardiac output.

Noradrenaline (norepinephrine)

Noradrenaline acts predominantly at α-adrenoceptors producing vasoconstriction. It is, therefore, indicated in the management of septic shock when hypotension (due to peripheral vasodilatation) persists despite adequate volume replacement.

Intra-aortic balloon counterpulsation

The intra-aortic balloon pump (IABP) is a mechanical device used to augment the cardiac output (Table 1.5).

Table 1.5: Uses of the Intra-aortic balloon pump (IABP).

Insertion	Positioned in the descending thoracic aorta distal to the origin of the left subclavian artery via a transfemoral insertion
Mechanism of action	Balloon inflates in diastole and deflates in systole, resulting in an increase in both diastolic and mean arterial pressure and, hence, coronary perfusion pressure, but a reduction in afterload
Indications	Potentially correctable mechanical cause for cardiogenic shock (e.g. acute mitral regurgitation or ventricular septal defect complicating myocardial infarction)
Complications	Lower limb ischaemia (requires removal of the IABP), balloon rupture, balloon entrapment, haematoma and infection

Management of atrial fibrillation (AF)

- Treat underlying cause, e.g. postoperative complications such as chest infection, pulmonary embolism, acid–base or electrolyte disturbance.

- Control of a rapid ventricular response rate may partly reverse the adverse haemodynamic effects associated with AF.

  - drugs (in isolation or in combination) digoxin, β-blockers, diltiazem, verapamil and amiodarone.

  - DC cardioversion can be considered with a low risk of thrombo-embolism if the onset of AF was within 48 h.

Table 1.6: Summary of the optimisation of cardiac output in the critically ill patient.

Optimise preload	If hypovolaemic, replace fluids If volume overloaded, IV GTN and IV furosemide
Optimise afterload	Sodium nitroprusside or hydralazine
Indications for inotropes	Hypotension despite adequate filling pressures: Cardiogenic shock (dopamine and dobutamine) Septic shock (noradrenaline)
Indications for IABP	Acute mitral regurgitation or VSD
Treat AF	Control ventricular response rate Preserved LV function: β-blockers, verapamil, diltiazem Impaired LV function: digoxin, amiodarone DC cardioversion

Summary of the principles of cardiovascular physiology and pharmacology

Flow = pressure/resistance
Cardiac output = SBP/SVR
Therefore, SBP = (SV × HR) × SVR.

Systemic blood pressure can be regulated by manipulation of any of the factors above:

- SV relates to preload and the inotropic capability (contractility) of the heart, mediated by β_1-receptors.

- HR relates to the chronotropic activity of the heart and is mediated by β_1-receptors.

- SVR relates to afterload and is related to α_1-receptors.

Other commonly used cardiovascular drugs

- Digoxin:

  - Use: ventricular rate control in AF.

- Dose:

  - loading 250–500 µg IV over 30 min (repeated after 6 h if necessary).

  - maintenance 62.5–250 µg day^{-1} depending on renal function.

- S/E:

  - GIT: anorexia, nausea and vomiting, diarrhoea, abdominal pain.

  - CNS: headache, visual disturbance.

  - CVS: arrhythmias, heart block.

  - toxicity: more likely in presence of hypokalaemia/renal failure.

- Amiodarone:

  - Use: most supraventricular and ventricular arrhythmias including AF, SVT, VT.

  - Dose:

    - IV loading 5 mg kg^{-1} over 1 h, followed by 15 mg kg^{-1} over next 23 h.

    - oral loading 600 mg every day for first week then 400 mg day^{-1} for second week 200 mg day^{-1} maintenance.

  - S/E:

    - corneal microdeposits.

    - phototoxic reactions.

    - thyroid dysfunction.

    - pneumonitis.

- Magnesium sulphate ($MgSO_4$):

  - Use:

    - cardiac tachyarrhythmias especially torsodes de pointes.

    - physiological antagonist to Ca^{2+}.

  - Dose:

    - aim for plasma level > 1 mmol l^{-1}.

    - 1 g = 2 ml 50% = 4 mmol.

    - typical dose 8 mmol over 20 mins followed by 60 mmol over 24 hours.

- S/E:

  - vasodilatation → hypotension.

  - muscle relaxation → respiratory dysfunction.

- Adenosine.

  - Use: chemical cardioversion of paroxysmal SVT.

  - Dose:

    - 3 mg followed by 6 mg, then 12 mg (if no effect).

    - given as a rapid bolus followed by a saline flush.

    - very short duration of action of a few seconds.

  - S/E:

    - bradycardia (may require temporary pacing).

    - vasodilatation → flushing + hypotension.

      chest pain.

    - bronchospasm.

CARDIAC ARREST AND RESUSCITATION

R Andrew Archbold

Classification of cardiac arrest

In cardiac arrest, the heart cannot maintain a cardiac output sufficient to generate a palpable pulse. There are three types, classified by the underlying heart rhythm:

- Ventricular tachycardia (VT) or ventricular fibrillation (VF).

- Asystole

- Pulseless electrical activity (PEA) } (non-VT/VF)

The management algorithm for asystole and PEA (formerly electromechanical dissociation, EMD) is the same. They are, therefore, grouped together as non-VT/VF.

Principles of management

Irreversible brain damage occurs within three minutes of circulatory arrest. Basic life support (BLS) aims to maintain cerebral oxygenation until defibrillation and advanced life support (ALS) can be initiated in an attempt to restore a cardiac output. The administration of a DC shock in pulseless VT/VF should be as early as possible because the chance of successful defibrillation decreases by 10% min⁻¹. These principles are encompassed in 'the chain of survival'.

Chain of survival

1 Call for help.

2 Basic life support.

3 Early defibrillation.

4 Advanced life support.

Basic life support (Table 1.7)

BLS is performed when no equipment or drugs are available. The principles encompass patient and rescuer safety, and assessment of the airway (and cervical spine), breathing and circulation (SSS, ABC).

- **S**afety.

- **S**hout at the patient.

- **S**hake the patient gently (take care when cervical spine injuries are possible). Is he unconscious; does he need your help?

- **A**irway (including cervical spine control): open airway, remove any visible obstruction. In trauma cases, maintain in line immobilisation of the cervical spine while securing the airway. If the airway is compromised, use chin lift or jaw thrust rather than head tilt.

- **B**reathing: examine patient for signs of respiratory effort and chest expansion. If no effective respiratory effort, send for or seek assistance if not already done. Turn patient onto his back and commence mouth to mouth ventilation with two initial rescue breaths.

- **C**irculation: examine patient for signs of a circulation (respiratory effort, swallowing, carotid pulse). If carotid pulse is present, continue rescue breathing and recheck pulse every minute. If no output in a witnessed arrest, administer a precordial thump (this is sometimes effective in reverting VT or VF to sinus rhythm). If this does not achieve a cardiac output, institute cardiac massage, applying downward pressure two-finger breadths superior to the xiphisternum.

Table 1.7: Recommended basic life support technique (2000).

Compressions:ventilations	15:2
Tidal volume	700–1000 ml over 1.5–2 s
Compression rate	100 min^{-1}
Compression depth	4–5 cm or one-third width of chest

Effective BLS achieves a cardiac output ~30% of that during sinus rhythm.

Advanced Life Support (Advanced Cardiac Life Support)

ALS describes resuscitation with the aid of drugs and equipment. The principles of ABC (maintaining the airway, assisting breathing and assisting the circulation) still apply.

VT or VF are the commonest cardiac rhythms to underlie cardiac arrest associated with heart disease. Management is aimed at the rapid administration of a DC shock.

Pulseless VT or VF (Figure 1.2)

If the rhythm changes to a non-VT/VF rhythm, DC shock is no longer indicated and the cardiac arrest is managed as for non-VT/VF (see below).

Non-VT/VF (Figure 1.2)

Non-VT/VF rhythms (PEA and asystole) carry a worse prognosis than VT/VF. Reversible causes should be sought and include: hypovolaemia, hypoxia, hypothermia, cardiac tamponade, tension pneumothorax, pulmonary embolus, hyperkalaemia, overdose with calcium blockers or β-adrenoceptor antagonists.

Cardiac arrest in trauma

The principles of resuscitation remain 'ABC', but cervical injury is more common and must be formally excluded. Reversible causes of cardiac arrest after trauma that should be considered include hypovolaemia due to haemorrhage (visible or concealed in the chest or abdomen), tension pneumothorax and cardiac tamponade.

Cross-reference

Chapter 1, p. 7.   CSiG

Further reading

ILCOR Advisory Statements: Single-rescuer adult basic life support. An advisory statement from the Basic Life Support Working Group of the International Liaison Committee on Resuscitation. *Circulation* 1997; 95: 2174–9.

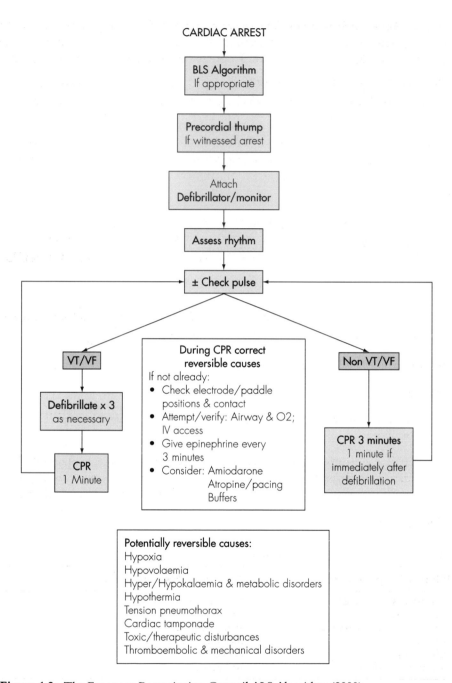

Figure 1.2: The European Resuscitation Council ALS Algorithm (2000).

ILCOR Advisory Statements: The universal advanced life support algorithm. An advisory statement from the Advanced Life Support Working Group of the International Liaison Committee on Resuscitation. *Circulation* 1997; 95: 2180–2.

The 1998 European Resuscitation Council guidelines for adult single rescuer basic life support. Basic Life Support Working Group of the European Resuscitation Council. *British Medical Journal* 1998; 316: 1870–6.

The 1998 European Resuscitation Council guidelines for adult advanced life support. Advanced Life Support Working Group of the European Resuscitation Council. *British Medical Journal* 1998; 316: 1863–9.

CLINICAL ASSESSMENT AND INVASIVE MONITORING OF VOLUME STATUS, CARDIAC OUTPUT AND SYSTEMIC VASCULAR RESISTANCE

R Andrew Archbold

The accurate assessment of volume status and cardiovascular haemodynamics is central to the appropriate management of the critically ill patient.

Assessment of volume status

History

- **Hypovolaemia:** haemorrhage, haematemesis, diarrhoea, vomiting or anorexia.

- **Volume overload:** history of heart failure, valvular disease, myocardial infarction, hypertension or diabetes mellitus. Breathlessness, paroxysmal nocturnal dyspnoea or oedema may be attributable to heart failure.

Examination

Table 1.8: Assessment of volume status.

Signs of hypovolaemia	Signs of volume overload
Dry mucous membranes	Tachycardia
Tachycardia	Raised JVP
Postural or frank hypotension	Third heart sound
Invisible JVP	Lung crepitations
Clear lung fields	Oedema
Absence of oedema	Tachypnoea

Urine output and fluid balance

- Oliguria (see Chapter 3) → early sign of either hypovolaemia or cardiogenic shock. Not helpful in the differential diagnosis of shock, but indicates the need for a prompt assessment of volume status and initiation of appropriate treatment.

- Fluid balance charts may provide evidence of inadequate fluid replacement in a patient who is nil by mouth, or who has excessive nasogastric, stoma or drain losses. Conversely, a large positive balance might explain the development of heart failure.

Chest X-ray (Figure 1.3)

The identification of pulmonary oedema (see Pulmonary oedema) (in the presence of raised filling pressures) confirms volume overload and the need for preload reduction and diuretics. The absence of pulmonary oedema is also an important finding, allowing the administration of a fluid challenge to the hypotensive or oliguric patient.

Table 1.9: Clinical assessment of volume status in the hypotensive or oliguric patient.

	Hypovolaemia	Volume overload
History	Volume loss or poor intake	Known heart failure or suggestive history
Examination	Postural hypotension, JVP↓, clear lungs, no oedema	JVP↑, third heart sound, crepitations, oedema
Fluid balance	Negative	Positive
CXR	No pulmonary oedema	Pulmonary oedema

Invasive monitoring is indicated when volume status remains uncertain after clinical evaluation. It can also be used to guide fluid administration in patients who are at risk of volume overload such as the elderly or those with a history of heart disease.

Central venous pressure (CVP) monitoring

The CVP represents the preload or filling pressure of the right side of the heart. It can be measured by the connection of a manometer or pressure transducer to a cannula within the internal jugular or subclavian vein. The CVP equates to the height of a column of fluid that is supported by the venous circulation.

- Normal range is 5–12 mmHg.

- Low CVP indicates hypovolaemia.

- High CVP usually indicates volume overload.

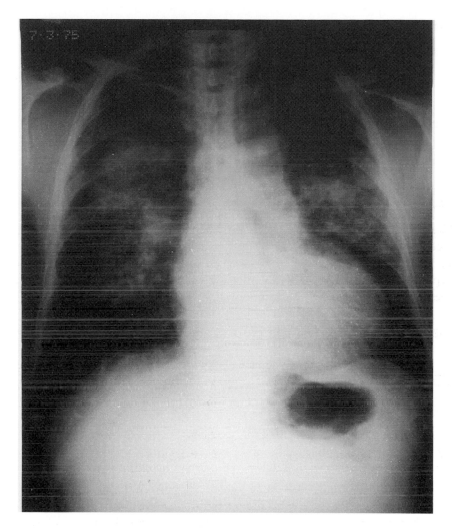

Figure 1.3: PA chest radiograph showing peri-hilar alveolar shadowing. In addition, the heart size is at the upper limit of normal. These are the signs of acute pulmonary oedema ('bat's wing' shadowing).

- If there is disparity between the function of the right and left ventricle (e.g. right ventricular infarction, pulmonary embolism, cor-pulmonale, left ventricular disease), however, the filling pressure of the right heart (CVP) may not reflect the filling pressure of the left heart. In these circumstances, the CVP will not be an accurate guide to volume status and measurement of the pulmonary artery occlusion pressure (PAOP) is indicated.

Pulmonary artery catheterisation (Figure 1.4 and Tables 1.10–12)

Pulmonary artery occlusion pressure monitoring

PAOP is an indirect measure of left atrial pressure and, hence, the preload or fill-ing pressure of the left heart. It is measured using a Pulmonary Artery Flotation Catheter (see Chapter 6, Pulmonary Artery Flotation Catheter), which contains a pressure transducer at its tip distal to an inflatable balloon (Figure 1.4). The resist-ance within the pulmonary veins is low so PAOP reflects left atrial pressure. If the catheter cannot be 'wedged' to obtain a PAOP trace, the pulmonary artery end-diastolic pressure is a useful measure of left ventricular filling pressure.

Table 1.10: Interpretation of PAOP.

PAOP	mmHg	Clinical situation
Normal	8–12	
Low	< 5	Hypovolaemia
Low with pulmonary oedema		ARDS
High	> 18	Volume overload

Measures of cardiac output

Objective measures of cardiac output are useful in the diagnosis and management of shock (Table 1.12) in which they can be used to guide inotropic therapy.

Thermodilution

The most commonly used method for the determination of cardiac output in the HDU/ITU setting is thermodilution. A known volume (typically 10 ml) of cold crystalloid is injected into the right atrial port of a Pulmonary Artery Flotation Catheter. A thermistor at the catheter tip measures the resultant transient temper-ature decrease in the pulmonary artery. The area under the curve when fall in tem-perature is plotted against time correlates with cardiac output, which is calculated by computer.

Oesophageal Doppler

The oesophageal Doppler monitor measures velocity of blood flow within the descending thoracic aorta. The area within the velocity–time waveform (velocity time integral) multiplied by the aortic cross-sectional area (obtained from a nomo-gram based upon age, height and weight) is the aortic blood flow from which stroke volume and cardiac output can be derived. This data can also be used to extrapolate information on volume status, SVR and myocardial contractility.

Echocardiography

Transthoracic echocardiography is a non-invasive method of assessing ventricular function and by implication cardiac output (see Electrocardiography and echocardiography in the surgical patient).

Systemic vascular resistance (SVR)

SVR can be calculated from aortic pressure, right atrial pressure and cardiac output.

SVR = 80 (mean aortic pressure – mean right atrial pressure)/cardiac output.

The determination of SVR is helpful in the diagnosis of critically ill patients (table 1.12) and repeated measurements can be used to monitor the effects of fluid and inotropic therapy.

Table 1.11: Indications for pulmonary artery catheterisation.

Measurement of PAOP to determine volume status and optimise cardiac output:
- Oliguria
- Hypotension
- RV infarction
- Cardiogenic shock
- Septic shock
- ARDS

Measurement of cardiac output/SVR to guide inotropic therapy:
- Cardiogenic shock
- Septic shock

Measurement of right heart blood O_2 saturations:
- Diagnosis of left to right shunt (VSD)
- Mixed venous (PA) O_2 concentration needed for some measures of cardiac output

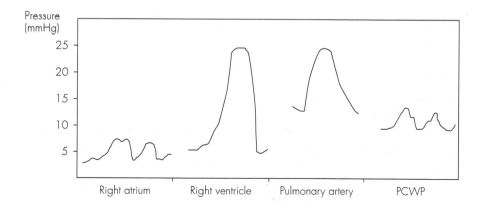

Figure 1.4: Pressure traces obtained from a pulmonary artery catheter.

Table 1.12: Differential diagnosis of shock using haemodynamic parameters from pulmonary artery flotation catheterisation.

	PAOP	Cardiac output	SVR
Hypovolaemia	↓	↓	↑
Cardiogenic shock	↑	↓	↑
Septic shock	↓	↑	↓

PAOP, pulmonary artery occlusion pressure; SVR, systemic vascular resistance.

Cross-reference

Chapter 37, p. 356.

Stoker MR. Preoperative management of cardiovascular disease.   SURGERY
Surgery 1999: 17; 87–91.

Further reading

Davidson CJ, Fishman RF, Bonow RO. Cardiac catheterisation. In Braunwald E (ed.), *Heart Disease: A Textbook of Cardiovascular Medicine* 5th ed (Philadelphia: W. B. Saunders 1997).

SPECIAL INVESTIGATIONS: ELECTROCARDIO-GRAPHY AND ECHOCARDIOGRAPHY IN THE SURGICAL PATIENT

R Andrew Archbold

Electrocardiography (ECG)

Atrial fibrillation (see Cardiac output: physiology and pharmacology)

ECG features (Figure 1.5):

1   absence of P-waves.

2   irregularity of the ventricular (QRS) response.

- AF occurs in ~5% of subjects aged 70–80 years and in ~10% of those with clinical evidence of cardiovascular disease, e.g. ischaemic heart disease, valve disease or hypertension.

- AF is also a frequent postoperative complication, occurring after 20–40% of CABG operations, for instance, when it is associated with increased morbidity, prolongation of hospital stay and an increased use of resources.

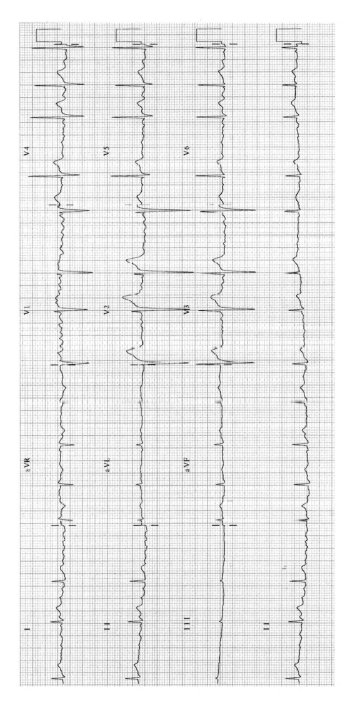

Figure 1.5: Atrial Fibrillation (AF).

Pulmonary embolism

ECG changes:

1 Most common is sinus tachycardia.

2 AF.

3 Right bundle branch block.

4 Right axis deviation.

5 Classical 'S1Q3T3' (S-wave in lead I, Q-wave in lead III and T-wave inversion in lead III) is seen only rarely.

The diagnosis should be suspected, particularly in the postoperative period, in the patient who presents with chest pain, dyspnoea, hypotension or hypoxia.

Myocardial infarction (MI)

ECG (Figure 1.6):

1 May be normal or only minor changes.

2 Characteristically gives rise to ST segment elevation.

Acute MI (AMI) is well recognised as one of the 'medical' causes of abdominal pain and may arise as a postoperative complication so it is important that ischaemic ECG changes can be interpreted. Thrombolysis is contraindicated in the early postoperative period.

Hyperkalaemia

Characteristic ECG changes (Figure 1.7):

1 Peaked T-waves.

2 Broadening of the QRS complex.

3 Reduction in P-wave amplitude.

Most commonly seen in acute renal failure, there is no absolute threshold of potassium concentration above which these changes occur. Nevertheless, the presence of ECG changes and/or a plasma potassium concentration > 6.5 mmol l^{-1} indicates the need for urgent treatment.

Transthoracic echocardiography (TTE)

TTE allows non-invasive, real-time imaging at the bedside, which makes it ideal for assessment in the critically ill, and provides information regarding cardiac structure, function and haemodynamics (Table 1.13).

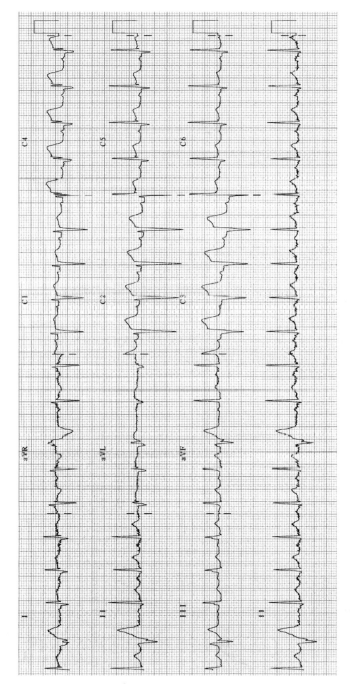

Figure 1.6: ECG of acute anterior myocardial infarction. There is ST elevation in leads V_{2-5} and Q-waves in leads V_{3-5}.

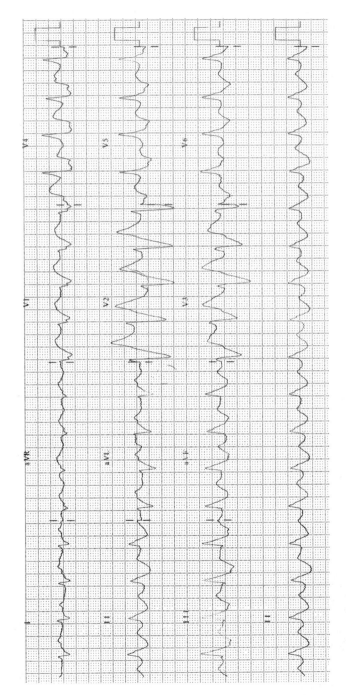

Figure 1.7: ECG of hyperkalaemia.

Table 1.13: Indications for TTE in the surgical patient.

General indications	Specific indications
Pre-operative risk stratification	Congenital heart disease
Peri-operative monitoring	Valvular disease
Diagnosis of the critically ill patient	Infective endocarditis
	Left ventricular disease
	Pericardial effusion (Figure 1.8)
	Aortic dissection (Figure 1.9)
	Intracardiac shunts
	Pulmonary embolism

Specific clinical scenarios

- The hypotensive patient: used to differentiate between:

  - cardiogenic shock (dilated, hypokinetic left ventricle).

  - cardiac tamponade (pericardial effusion with right ventricular diastolic collapse).

  - PE (dilated right ventricle with paradoxical septal motion).

- The post-AMI patient with cardiovascular collapse: used to diagnose the potentially correctable causes.

  - acute mitral regurgitation due to papillary muscle rupture.

  - VSD due to rupture of the interventricular septum.

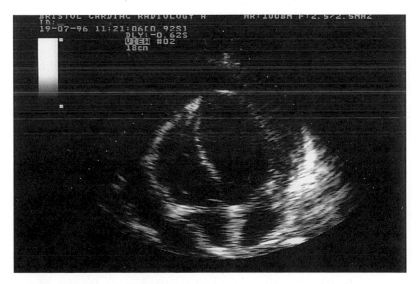

Figure 1.8: Large pericardial effusion. Note that the fluid does not extend behind the left atrium as there is no pericardial space in this area (Reproduced from Practical Echocardiography, GMM, 1999).

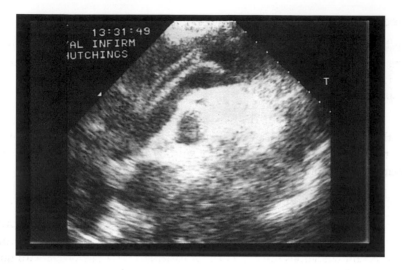

Figure 1.9: Suprasternal image of a dissection in the ascending aorta showing a complex intimal flap, which was very mobile on the real-time scan (Reproduced from Practical Echocardiography, GMM, 1999).

Table 1.14: Indications for transoesophageal echocardiography.

Inadequate TTE images
Valvular disease (prosthetic and native)
Endocarditis (diagnosis and complications)
Cardiac source of embolus
Aortic pathology (dissection, aneurysm, atheroma)
Congenital heart disease (especially ASD)
Intra-operative monitoring of LV function and assessment of operative results
Chest trauma

- In aortic dissection, the dissection flap can sometimes be visualised in the aortic root. Supportive evidence for the diagnosis may be obtained from the presence of a pericardial effusion or aortic regurgitation.

Limitations

- Image quality is often suboptimal in obese patients or those with COAD.

- Standard TTE views may not be possible after sternotomy, thoracotomy or chest trauma.

- Evaluation of prosthetic valves by TTE is difficult because of echo reverberations and shadowing generated by the echo-reflective material within the valve.

Transoesophageal echocardiography (TOE)

TOE is less widely available than TTE and is semi-invasive. Nevertheless, it is safe carrying a mortality of 1 in 10 000. Oesophageal pathology such as stricture or varices is the only absolute contraindication (Table 1.14).

Endocarditis

TOE is superior to TTE for the detection of vegetations (Figure 1.11), and, hence, the diagnosis of endocarditis. It is able to define complications of endocarditis that require surgical treatment, e.g. aortic root abscess and prosthetic paravalvular regurgitation.

Source of embolus

TOE has a far higher sensitivity for the detection of potential sources of cardiac embolism such as left atrial thrombus, patent foramen ovale or aortic atheroma. Current recommendations reserve TOE for patients < 50 years of age with unexplained embolism or if endocarditis, myxoma or aortic dissection is suspected.

Aortic dissection

This can be diagnosed by TOE (in experienced hands) as accurately as MRI and CT scanning, both of which may also pose practical problems for the imaging of critically ill patients. TOE provides additional information regarding aortic valve and left ventricular function and the relationship between the dissection flap and the coronary artery ostea.

Trauma

Traumatic rupture of the aorta is usually caused by a deceleration injury, typically a road traffic accident. If not immediately fatal, the diagnosis can be made by TOE. Additional information after trauma regarding the presence of a pericardial effusion or regional hypokinesia indicating contusion or infarction can be sought. TOE may also be useful after penetrating chest injury to assess the integrity of the heart and great vessels.

Intra-operative TOE

TOE is widely used in the US for the peri-operative assessment of volume status and cardiac function:

- A contracted hyperdynamic left ventricle in the setting of hypotension would suggest hypovolaemia and the need for fluid administration.

- The observation of new regional akinesia after CABG surgery would suggest graft occlusion and the need for graft revision.

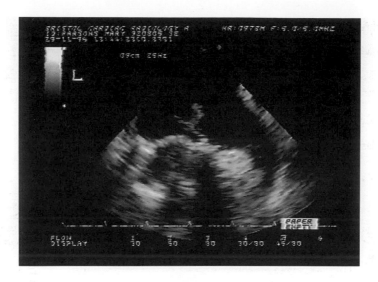

Figure 1.10: Infective vegetation on a mechanical mitral valve. In systole, with the valve closed, a highly mobile vegetation can be seen arising from the atrial side of the sewing ring (Reproduced from Practical Echocardiography, GMM 1999).

- TOE plays a major role in determining whether the regurgitant mitral valve is repairable. At the conclusion of the repair, the operative result can be assessed and the repair modified if significant regurgitation remains.

- The hypotensive patient early after cardiac surgery is a common clinical scenario (see Postoperative complications of cardiothoracic surgery). An important diagnosis to consider is right heart compression by localised clot. This is often not visible on TTE, but can be seen on TOE and it requires surgical evacuation.

Cross-reference

Chapter 37, p. 356.   CSiG

Madden BP. Assessment of cardiac and pulmonary function. *Surgery* 1999; 17: iii–vi.

SURGERY

Further reading

Chambers JB, de Belder MA, Moore D. Echocardiography in stroke and transient ischaemic attack. *Heart* 1997; 78 (suppl. 1), 2–6.

Treasure T, Brecker S. The role of echocardiography in the diagnosis of aortic dissection. *Journal of Heart Valve Disease* 1996; 5: 623–9.

MANAGEMENT OF HAEMORRHAGE AND SHOCK

Definition

Shock is a state in which tissue perfusion and oxygenation are inadequate to maintain organ function and leads to reversible and if prolonged irreversible organ damage.

Classification

Baue classified shock into the following categories (Table 1.15):

Table 1.15: Classification of Shock (Baue).

Hypovolaemia	Tissue injury	Cardiogenic	Septic	Vasoactive
Bleeding	Trauma	Intrinsic (MI)		Spinal
Burns	Operation	Extrinsic (PE, tamponade)		Anaphylactic
Intestinal	Inflammatory			
obstruction	Response			
Dehydration	Volume loss			

Diagnosis

- Tachycardia: sympathetic stimulation.
- Poor organ perfusion:
  - cold, clammy, confused.
  - ↓ urine output.

Causes

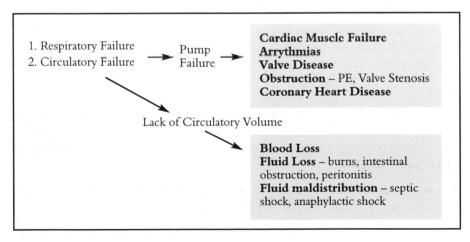

Figure 1.11: Causes of shock.

Pathophysiology

Ischaemia and impaired tissue perfusion → generalised cellular damage → anaerobic metabolism:

- → decreased ATP formation.

- → lactic acid formation → metabolic acidosis.

Decreased ATP →

- Failure Na^+/K^+ pump.

- Na^+ H_2O influx.

- Cellular swelling → impaired function.

Clinical

Clinical features vary for the different types of shock (Table 1.16).

Table 1.16: Clinical features of shock.

	Hypovolaemic/cardiogenic	Septic
Pulse rate	↑	bounding ↑
Blood pressure	↓	normal/↑
Peripheries	cold and clammy	febrile and pink
Respiratory rate	↑	↑
Urine output	↓	↓

Hypovolaemic shock can be further classified by the severity of blood loss, and the symptoms vary with severity (Table 1.17).

Table 1.17: Symptoms of hypovolaemic shock.

	I	II	III	IV
Blood loss (%)	10–15	15–30	30–40	> 40
Blood loss (litres)	0.75	0.8–1.5	1.5–2.0	> 2.0
Heart rate (beats min⁻¹)*	normal	normal/↑	↑ (> 120)	↑
Blood pressure*	normal	↓ (postural)	↓	↓↓↓
Urine output (ml h⁻¹)	normal > 30	↓ 20–30	↓ < 20	nil
Respiratory rate (breaths min⁻¹)	normal	normal	↑ (> 20)	↑↑ (> 20)
Mental state	alert	anxious	confused	comatose

*Compensation for hypovolaemia initially by ↑ heart rate to maintain cardiac output and BP.

Treatment

The aim of treatment is resuscitation (ABC) and the maximisation of oxygen delivery to the tissues (see Chapter 3: Multisystem failure).

The four key principles are:

- Ventilation and oxygenation.
- Volume resuscitation (fluid used = fluid lost).
- Pulmonary support.
- Cardiac support.

Monitoring

- Pulse, blood pressure, respiratory rate, urine output, temperature.
- CVP, PAOP, ABG, electrolytes, acid–base, renal and liver function.
- Glucose, clotting, haemoglobin.
- Mental state.

Complications

- SIRS, MODS and multi organ failure (see Chapter 3, Multisystem fail ure and systemic inflammatory response syndrome).
- Acute renal failure (see Chapter 3, Renal failure: diagnosis of renal failure, complications of renal failure): acute tubular necrosis if hypovolaemia persists.
- Adult respiratory distress syndrome (see Chapter 2, ARDS).
- GI complications.
  - stress ulceration.
  - bacteraemia and sepsis.

Prognosis

- Depends on underlying cause, severity and duration.
- Maintenance of cardiac output and oxygen delivery are associated with improved survival.
- Increasing age and pre-existing medical conditions adversely affect survival.
- Cardiogenic shock: 80% mortality.

- Hypovolaemic shock:

  - prognosis related to the nature of the underlying problem.

  - excellent prognosis with early aggressive resuscitation.

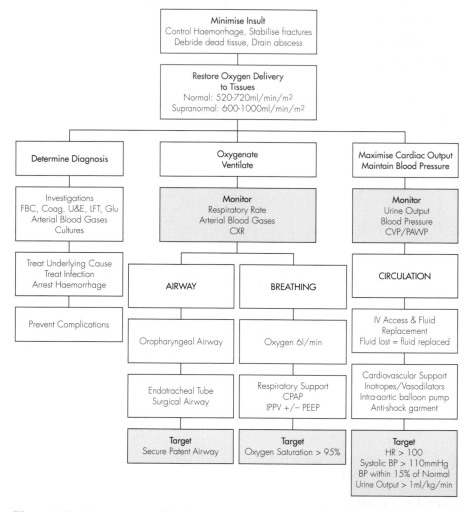

Figure 1.12: Management of shock.

Cross-reference

Chapter 37, p. 355. CSiG

Ginolami A, Greenstein AS, Little RA Shock. *Surgery* 1998: 16; SURGERY
187–9.

PULMONARY OEDEMA

Pulmonary oedema is the result of increased interstitial fluid in the lungs. The general causes can be divided into three categories:

- Neurogenic, which is caused by overwhelming sympathetic stimulation as a result of ↑ ICP.

- Increased capillary permeability, e.g. ARDS.

- Cardiogenic (see below).

Causes

- Myocardial infarction/ischaemia.

- Valve disease, e.g. mitral stenosis/regurgitation, aortic regurgitation.

- Arrhythmias.

- Cardiomyopathy.

- Sepsis.

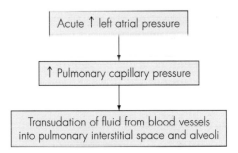

Figure 1.13: Pathophysiology of pulmonary oedema.

Pathophysiology

Clinical symptoms

- Dyspnoea, tachypnoea.

- Anxiety (feeling of impending doom).

- ↑ Sympathetic drive

    - tachycardia.

- peripheral vasoconstriction (cold).

- sweating (clammy).

- Cough productive of pink frothy sputum (blood staining).

Clinical signs

- Wheeze.

- Fine inspiratory crackles heard throughout lungfields.

- Gallop rhythm (third heart sound).

Investigations

- ECG:
    - left ventricular hypertrophy and strain.
    - myocardial infarction or ischaemia.
    - arrhythmias.
- ABG:
    - ↓ PaO_2.
    - ↓ $PaCO_2$ initially, then ↑ $PaCO_2$ due to impaired gas exchange.
- CXR (Figure 1.3):
    - distension of upper lobe veins →↑ pulmonary venous pressure.
    - bilateral perihilar shadowing (also known as bat's wing or butterfly shadowing) → represents alveolar fluid.
    - Kerley B lines → represents interstitial oedema.
    - pleural effusion.
    - may be cardiomegaly.

Management

The aim of treatment is to:

- ↓ Preload (to ↓ myocardial distension).

- ↓ Afterload (to ↓ myocardial work).

1 Sit up.

2 High concentration oxygen by facemask (reservoir bag).

3 Opioids (incremental IV morphine 1–2 mg boluses, up to 10 mg). This relieves anxiety and provides a degree of vasodilatation.

4   Diuretics (furosemide 40–80 mg IV). This initially vasodilates and later reduces intravascular fluid volume.

5   Nitrates (GTN) (Table 1.4). This is a potent vasodilator.

If there is no improvement with these measures, the patient may need other interventions:

→   Inotropic support (with an inodilator such as dobutamine or dopexamine) (Table 1.5).

→   Mechanical ventilation ($\downarrow$ compliance requires the use of PEEP to improve oxygenation).

Co-existing hypertension, ischaemia and arrhythmias should be treated as necessary.

Monitoring

- Continuous ECG.
- NIBP (cycling at 3–5-min intervals): may need invasive BP.
- Pulse oximeter.
- Regular ABG.

GENERAL PRINCIPLES OF CARDIOPULMONARY BYPASS

Indications

- Repair intracardiac defects.
- Repair or replace cardiac valves.
- Coronary artery bypass grafting.
- Supradiaphragmatic aortic operations.
- Heart/heart–lung transplantation.
- Cardiac support.
- Pulmonary support.
- Hypothermia.

Technique

The patient should be anticoagulated with heparin 300 u kg^{-1}.

After cannulation of the atrium and ascending aorta, blood is drained from the patient by gravity. It passes through the oxygenator (Figure 1.14) and is returned via the cannula in the ascending aorta

Increasing the bypass time can result in increased end organ damage.

Complications

- Haematological:
    - coagulation: resulting in decreased platelets and fibrinogen.
    - red blood cell trauma: haemoglobinaemia and haemoglobinuria.
- bleeding resulting from activation and loss of platelets or failure to neutralise heparin.
- Diffuse inflammatory reaction resulting from activation of complement.
- Air micro-embolism.
- Psychiatric disturbances and cerebral dysfunction.
- ARDS (see Chapter 2).

Cross-reference CSiG

Chapter 9, p. 109.

Anderson J, Murday A, Mascaro J. Artificial circulations. SURGERY
Surgery 1994; 12: 137–40.

ANAEMIA AND TRANSFUSION

Anaemia

Definition

- Adult male: haemoglobin < 13.5 g dl^{-1}.
- Adult female: haemoglobin < 11.5 g dl^{-1}.
- Child 3 months to puberty: haemoglobin < 11.0 g dl^{-1}.
- At birth: haemoglobin < 15.0 g dl^{-1}.

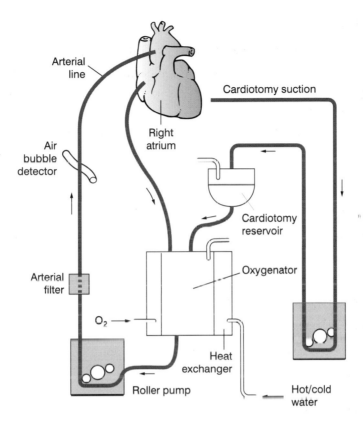

Figure 1.14: Components of a standard cardiopulmonary bypass circuit. Heat exchanger: utilised to decrease the metabolic rate: mild hypothermia (25–28°C). Deep hypothermia (18–20°C) employed to allow interruption of bypass (circulatory arrest). Oxygenator (three types): (1) bubble: O_2/N_2 mixture bubbled through blood; (2) membrane: oxygenation and CO_2 removal over a semipermeable membrane; and (3) microporous: gas exchange through pores in a polyethylene membrane. Reservoir: contains venous blood and also blood from the operative field; capacity >6 litres. Roller pump: flow rate between 2.4 and 2.8 1 m^{-2} min^{-1} to provide adequate perfusion and oxygenation. Filter: pore size usually 40 μm (Reproduced from Surgery Facts & Figures GMM 2000).

Classification

- By red cell indices (Table 1.18).

- By mechanism: decreased red cell production:

  - iron deficiency.

  - B$_{12}$/folate deficiency.

  - marrow failure.

- Abnormal red cell maturation: myelodysplasia.

- Increased red cell destruction:
    - auto-immune haemolytic anaemia.
    - Disseminated Intravascular Coagulopathy (see Disseminated intravascular coagulopathy).
- Other organ disease:
    - anaemia of chronic disease.
    - chronic renal failure.

Diagnosis

On full blood count, haemoglobin as per definition.

Table 1.18: Classification of anaemia by red cell indices.

	Microcytic hypochromic	Macrocytic	Normocytic normochromic
MCV (fl)	< 80	> 95	80–95
MCH (pg)	< 27		> 26
Diagnoses	Iron deficiency, thalassaemia	B$_{12}$/folate deficiency, liver disease	haemolysis, secondary anaemia, bone marrow failure

Clinical investigations

- WBC and platelets: is there a pancytopenia?
- Reticulocytes: ↑ in anaemia.
- Film: abnormal red cell morphology, e.g. dimorphic population.
- Bone marrow sample: aspiration or trephine.

Clinical treatment

- Treat underlying cause.
- Appropriate replacement therapy:
    - iron (ferrous sulphate) for iron deficiency anaemia.
    - B$_{12}$/folate as appropriate for megaloblastic anaemia.
- Transfuse as necessary.

Transfusion

Definition

Infusion of whole blood/blood component(s) from donor to recipient.

Pathophysiology

Compatibility needs to be ensured to avoid potentially fatal haemolytic reactions.

There are multiple blood group systems, the commonest being ABO (Table 1.19) and Rhesus. For details of others, see Further reading on p41.

Blood products and uses (Table 1.20)

Complications

- Immune:

    - Haemolytic Transfusion Reactions: ABO incompatibility.

    - Non-haemolytic febrile transfusion reactions: granulocyte specific antibodies.

Table 1.19: ABO blood groups.

Phenotype	Genotype	Antigen	Antibody	UK frequency (%)
O*	OO	O	anti-A, anti-B	46
A	AA/AO	A	anti-B	42
B	BB/BO	B	anti-A	9
AB**	AB	AB		3

*Universal donor; **universal recipient.

Table 1.20: Blood products and their uses.

Blood product	Dose	Use
Whole blood*	1 u = 450 ml	acute blood loss
Packed red cells*	300 ml	chronic anaemia
Red cell substitutes		experimental
Granulocyte concentrates*		severe neutropenia
Platelet concentrates*	6 u = 3 × 10¹⁰ platelets	severe thrombocytopenia with established bleeding/prophylaxis
Fresh frozen plasma (FFP)*	300 ml	replacement of coagulation factors
Human albumin 4.5%*		shock
Human albumin 20%		severe hypo-albuminaemia
Cryoprecipitate	10 iu	replacement in haemophilia A and von Willebrand's disease
Freeze-dried factor VIII		replacement in haemophilia A and von Willebrand's disease
Freeze-dried factor IX		replacement in Christmas disease
Immunoglobulin	1–2 g kg⁻¹	hypogammaglobulinaemia, immune thrombocytopenia

*Commonly used in critical care.

- Transmission of infection:

  - bacterial: syphilis.

  - protozoal: malaria, toxoplasmosis.

  - viral: cytomegalovirus, Epstein–Barr, HIV I and II, HTLV I and II, hepatitis, yellow fever.

Massive transfusion

Definitions

- Absolute: transfusion replacement of one or more times the body's blood volume within 24 h.
- Relative: transfusion rate of > 2 units h^{-1} for 2 h.

Pathophysiology

The platelet count in stored blood (at 4°C) is reduced through clumping after 24 h. There is further loss of coagulation factors V and VIII over the subsequent few days.

Clinical

Patients receiving massive transfusions often show abnormal bleeding. There are three main reasons for this:

- Dilutional thrombocytopenia.
- Impairment of platelet function.
- Loss of coagulation factors.

These defects can be minimised by the use of specific replacement factors:

- 2 units FFP
- 5 units platelets

for every 8–10 units of blood transfused.

Monitoring

Patients receiving massive transfusions require close monitoring of:

- FBC.
- Coagulation studies.
- U&E.
- Acid–base balance.

Complications of transfusion

- Thrombocytopenia.
- Coagulation factor depletion.
- Hypothermia (use blood warmers where possible).
- Hypocalcaemia.
- Hyperkalaemia.
- Acid–base disturbances.
- Oxygen affinity changes.
- SIRS (see Chapter 3, Multisystem failure and systemic inflammatory response syndrome).
- ARDS (see Chapter 2, ARDS).

Cross-reference

Chapter 9, p. 100.   CSiG

Stanworth SJ, Williamson LM. Blood transfusion in surgery.   SURGERY
Surgery 2000; 18: 48–52.

Huntly BJP, Rawlinson S. Blood transfusion. *Surgery* 1999; 17: 44–47.

SURGERY

Further reading

Hoffbrand AV, Pettit JE. *Essential Haematology*, 3rd edn (London: Blackwell Science, 1992).

SURGICAL BLEEDING

A bloodless operating field facilitates surgical dissection and enhances recovery.

Blood has a number of surgically important functions:

- Oxygen carriage: red cells and haemoglobin.
- Haemostasis: endothelial cells and platelets.
- Inflammatory response.
- Immunity.

Patients who are of concern with regard to bleeding are:

- Patients deficient in one or more blood components.
- Patients on anticoagulants.
- Patients who undergo massive bleeding.

There are a number of surgical implications in these patients (Table 1.21).

Table 1.21: Surgical implications of deficiency of blood components.

Condition	Implications
Anaemia	tissue hypoxia
↓ White cells	impaired inflammation and wound healing, prone to infection
Thrombocytopenia	bleeding

Table 1.22: Coagulation investigations.

Investigation	Measure of	Normal*	Uses	Examples
Blood count	platelet number and morphology	150–400 × 10^9 litre^{-1}		
Bleeding time	platelet plug formation *in vivo* (primary haemostasis)	3–10 min	disorders of platelet function. **Little use as screening test**	aspirin (↑). Collagen disorders (↑)
Activated partial thromboplastin time (APTT)	intrinsic and common pathways	30–50 s	monitoring heparin Rx. **Little use as screening test**	heparin (↑). Haemophilia A (↑)
Prothrombin time (PT)	extrinsic and common pathways	16–18 s	monitoring oral anticoagulant Rx. Assess liver. Detect vitamin K deficiency. **Little use as screening test**	warfarin (↑)
International Normalised Ratio (INR)	standardised PT	2.5–4.8 therapeutic levels	monitoring oral anticoagulant Rx	warfarin (↑)
Thrombin time (TT)	assesses conversion of fibrinogen to fibrin	12 s	diagnosis of DIC. Detects heparin if unexplained ↑ in APTT	DIC (↑)
Activated clotting time (ACT)	intrinsic pathway	*	quick assessment of coagulation state in ICU/ cardiac theatre	CPB (↑)
Fibrinogen degradation products (FDP)	assesses cleavage of fibrin and fibrinogen	< 10 mg ml^{-1}	diagnosis of DIC	DIC (↑)

* Local reference values should be used.

Table 1.23: Results of coagulation tests in common surgical scenarios.

	Platelets	PT	APTT	TT
DIC	↓	↑	↑	↑↑↑
Massive transfusion	↓	↑	↑	normal
Oral anticoagulants	normal	↑↑	↑	normal
Heparin	normal	↑	↑	↑

Pathophysiology

The response to surgery is a significant factor in surgical bleeding. Tissue injury results in the release of humoral mediators leading to a local inflammatory response. Use of a tourniquet or a clamp results in distal ischaemia and subsequent release of this can lead to reperfusion injury.

Clinical
Investigations

Major surgical bleeding should be investigated by full blood count and coagulation screening (prothrombin time (PT), activated partial thromboplastin time (APTT) and thrombin time (TT)) (Table 1.22). Other uses of these investigations are shown in Table 1.22.

Results of these tests for surgical bleeding problems are shown in Table 1.23.

Control of bleeding

Where surgical bleeding is a problem, there are a number of methods of gaining control of haemorrhage (Table 1.24).

Cross-reference
Chapters 9, p. 100, and 36, p. 351. CSiG

Haemostasis and bleeding problems. *Surgery* 1999; 17: v–vii. SURGERY

Further reading

Forbes CD, Cuschieri A. *Management of Bleeding Disorders in Surgical Practice* (Oxford: Blackwells, 1993).

Table 1.24: Methods of bleeding control.

Surgical methods of controlling massive haemorrhage	direct compression cross-clamping descending thoracic aorta for major vascular/organ injury insertion of a shunt
Surgical adjuncts	pressure packing: pelvic bleeding pneumatic anti-shock garment ligation of feeding vessels
Thermal methods	cautery/diathermy (monopolar and bipolar) photocoagulation
Non-thermal methods	balloon tamponade (Sengstaken–Blakemore tube) sclerosing agents tissue adhesives angiographic embolisation surgery
Pharmacological agents	desmopressin somatostatin tranexamic acid aprotinin

THROMBOTIC DISORDERS

Table 1.25: Arterial and venous thrombotic disorders.

	Arterial thrombi	**Venous thrombi**
Classification	occur at sites of damaged endothelial cells	occur due to Virchow's triad (stasis, altered flow, altered components)
Pathophysiology	develop in relation to platelet reaction and accumulation. Are a response to vessel wall damage	are as a result of the generation of thrombin in areas of retarded flow
Risk factors	family history, male sex, diabetes mellitus, gout, hyperlipidaemia, hypertension, thrombocytosis, smoking, myocardial and peripheral vascular disease, increased factor VII and fibrinogen	**Coagulation factors**: hereditary (antithrombin III deficiency, protein C/S deficiency, factor V Leiden, abnormal fibrinogen or plasminogen), oestrogen therapy, lupus anticoagulant, pregnancy and puerperium, abdominal or hip surgery, trauma, malignancy, myocardial infarction **Stasis**: cardiac failure, cerebrovascular accident, immobility, pelvic obstruction, nephrotic syndrome, dehydration, hyperviscosity states, polycythaemia, varicose veins, pregnancy **Unknown**: increasing age, obesity, sepsis

Definition

Thrombi are solid masses or plugs formed in the circulation from blood constituents (Table 1.25).

Clinical
Investigations

The following investigations should be undertaken for thrombotic states:

- FBC/ESR: ↑ haematocrit, ↑ WCC, ↑ platelets.
- Blood film: myeloproliferative disorders.
- APTT: ↓ with activated clotting factors.
- TT: ↑ = abnormal fibrinogen.
- Fibrinogen assay.
- Antithrombin III assay.
- Protein C and S assays.
- Factor V Leiden DNA analysis.

Prevention

Those at increased risk (pelvic/abdominal surgery, major trauma, previous history, pregnancy) require prophylactic measures. The majority of critically ill patients on ICU will, by definition, be at increased risk of thrombo-embolism. Prophylactic measures include.

- Graduated compression stockings.
- Pneumatic compression devices.
- Low-dose heparin/low molecular weight heparin.
- Anti-platelet drugs (aspirin).
- Low-dose warfarin.

Treatment and monitoring

Anticoagulation is indicated for venous thromboses. Its role is less certain in arterial thromboses (Table 1.26).

Inferior vena caval filters (Greenfield filter) can be inserted to reduce the risk of pulmonary embolism (Table 1.27).

Thrombolysis is appropriate for major proximal vein thromboses, surgical embolectomy only for life-threatening proximal thromboses following failure of medical management.

Table 1.26: Anticoagulation and thrombolysis.

Route	Drug	Action	Administration	Monitoring
IV/SC	heparin	activates antithrombin III	IV: 1000–2000 uh⁻¹ SC: 15000 ubd MWH: 5000 ud⁻¹	APTT: 1.5–2 × normal
Oral	warfarin	↓ activity of factors II, VII–X	10, 10(5), 5 mg loading dose; 3–9 mg titrated day⁻¹	INR: 2–2.5 prophylactic; 2–3 DVT/PE; 3–4.5 recurrent PE
IV	streptokinase	fibrinolysis	1.5 M u for MI	
Oral	aspirin	inhibits cyclo-oxygenase	75 mg od	

Table 1.27: Indications for IVC filter insertion.

Absolute indications
- Pulmonary embolism with contraindication to anticoagulation
- Recurrent pulmonary emboli despite adequate anticoagulation

Relative indications
- DVT with contraindication to anticoagulation
- Large proximal DVT ± free floating thrombus
- Following pulmonary embolectomy

Complications

Complications of DVT are most often due to proximal thrombi:

- Pulmonary embolism.

- Post-thrombotic syndrome (pain, swelling, dermatitis, ulceration) – as a result of high venous pressure.

- Recurrent thromboses.

Cross-reference
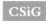

Chapter 36, p. 345.

Further reading

Donnelly R, London NJM (eds). *ABC of Arterial and Venous Disease* (London: British Medical Journal Publ. 2000).

Hoffbrand AV, Pettit JE. *Essential Haematology*, 3rd edn (Oxford: Blackwell Science, 1992).

DISSEMINATED INTRAVASCULAR COAGULOPATHY (DIC)

Definition

DIC is a dynamic condition of clotting activation and thrombin generation resulting in thrombosis and bleeding due to consumption of coagulation factors, fibrin deposition and fibrinolysis.

Causes

Over 100 identified. Most frequent causes:

- Sepsis.
- Shock and blood loss.
- Crush injuries.
- Head injury.
- Hypoxia.

Less common causes include:

- Obstetric complications.
- Burns.
- Transfusion reactions.
- Fat embolism.
- Malignancy.

Pathophysiology

Sudden release of thromboplastic material into the vascular system results in widespread deposition of fibrin in the microcirculation (with resultant consumption of fibrinogen).

Fibrin degradation products (FDP) are produced, further impairing coagulation.

The resultant effect is major bleeding and tissue ischaemia from the microvascular thrombi.

Clinical

Investigations

- Coagulation screen:
  - increased prothrombin time (PT).
  - increased activated partial thromboplastin time (APTT).

- increased thrombin time (TT).

- increased FDP.

- decreased fibrinogen.

- Haematology:

  - decreased platelets.

  - thrombocytopenia.

  - leucocytosis with left shift.

  - RBC fragments on microscopy.

Treatment

- Seek expert advice from a haematologist as this is a complex clinical condition.

- Haemodynamic support: blood product components: FFP, cryoprecipitate, platelets (see Anaemia and transfusion).

- Treat underlying cause:

  - antibiotics.

  - ERPC.

- Consider heparin (SC/IV) to cease intravascular coagulation and consumption of coagulative components.

Monitoring

Three to 6 h after treatment commences ($\downarrow\uparrow$ indicates the aim of treatment):

- FDP ($\downarrow$).

- Fibrinogen ($\uparrow$).

- Platelets ($\uparrow$).

- APTT ($\downarrow$).

- PT ($\downarrow$).

Complications

- Bleeding.

- Tissue ischaemia (see Pathophysiology).

Prognosis

The mortality rate of DIC is 65–85%, often due to the underlying condition.

Cross-reference
Chapter 9, p. 100.　CSiG

POSTOPERATIVE COMPLICATIONS OF CARDIOTHORACIC SURGERY

Timothy J. Jones

Surgery on the thoracic cavity is indicated in the treatment of a variety of conditions affecting the following organs and structures:

- Heart and great vessels.
- Lungs, mediastinum and parietal space.
- Oesophagus.
- Thymus.
- Diaphragm.
- Thoracic spine.

Pre-existing cardiac disease, operative trauma and the use of cardiopulmonary bypass (CPB) during cardiac surgery create specific postoperative problems. In common with all surgical complications the best practice is *prevention* by appropriate patient selection and good surgical technique.

The postoperative care of the majority of patients recovering from cardiothoracic surgery is uncomplicated. Once the patient is warm, haemodynamically stable with adequate respiratory function and no evidence of bleeding they are allowed to wake up before tracheal extubation. Whether this occurs in the operating room, recovery area or ITU is dependent upon the patient, operative procedure and unit protocol. To ensure that patients follow this uncomplicated course they need to be adequately monitored.

Monitoring (Tables 1.28 and 1.29)

Table 1.28: Postoperative monitoring.

Cardiovascular	heart rate	aim for sinus rhythm at 80–100 beats min⁻¹. Preoperative β-blockade may result in postoperative bradycardia
	blood pressure	hypotension prompts investigation and treatment
	CVP	indirect estimation of preload or right ventricular filling
	PAOP	provides an indirect measurement of left atrial pressure and preload. Also allows estimations of cardiac output
	left atrial pressure	provides accurate assessment of left-sided filling pressure. Used in severe left ventricular dysfunction, pulmonary hypertension or mechanical ventricular assist devices
Respiratory	airway pressure	positive pressure ventilation improves gas exchange and reduces the work of breathing
	oxygen saturation	aim for > 95%.
	ABG	enables decisions to be made about ventilation, extubation, physiotherapy, respiratory assistance or re-intubation
	CXR	position of IV catheters, chest drains and ET tube, atelectasis, pneumothoraces, pleural effusions, pulmonary oedema, pulmonary infiltrates and gastric dilatation
Haematology	blood loss	must be accurately monitored (Table 1.29)
	transfusion trigger	8 g dl⁻¹
	coagulation	treat abnormal results
Miscellaneous	urine output	indirect guide to CO (see Chapter 3, Oliguria)
	temperature	hypothermia due to heat loss from open thoracic cavity and hypothermic CPB
	acid–base balance	lactic acidaemia → metabolic acidosis
	glucose	hyperglycaemia secondary to surgical stress, adrenaline and corticosteroids
	analgesia	thoracic epidural for thoracotomy pain

Table 1.29: Indications for surgical exploration.

Bleeding:
- >500 ml h⁻¹
- >400 ml for 2 h
- >300 ml for 3 h

Evidence of cardiac tamponade

Complications
Cardiovascular
Arrhythmias

- Atrial arrhythmias, mainly atrial fibrillation (AF), occur in up to 30% of patients and are associated with increased mortality. This can result in reduced cardiac output because atrial systole contributes up to one-third of ventricular systole. The onset of AF should prompt:

  - examination.

  - optimisation of ABG and serum potassium/magnesium.

  - avoidance of high cardiac filling pressures.

  - haemodynamic compromise requires DC cardioversion.

  - otherwise chemical cardioversion with agents such as amiodarone or digoxin.

  - heparinisation should be considered due to the risk of embolisation from atrial thrombus.

- Sinus bradycardia may occur following cardiac surgery. Treatment is by pacing (epicardial or atrial) or pharmacological measures (atropine or isoprenaline).

- Ventricular arrhythmias: uncommon postoperatively and suggestive of myocardial ischaemia or damage (see Cardiac arrest and resuscitation).

- Conduction abnormalities and heart block: may occur after valvular heart surgery and CABG surgery using cold cardioplegia for myocardial protection, particularly in association with impaired LV function. These patients usually leave the operating theatre with atrial and ventricular temporary epicardial pacing wires. The type of heart block and ventricular rate dictate the need and mode of pacing.

Low cardiac output

The primary objective for patients recovering from thoracic surgery and particularly cardiac surgery is a satisfactory cardiac output (see Cardiac output: physiology and pharmacology). A cardiac index > 2.5 l min^{-1}m^{-2} with a heart rate < 100 beats min^{-1} with warm, well-perfused peripheries and good urine output is optimal.

The postoperative causes of low cardiac output are given in Table 1.30.

Making the diagnosis of low cardiac output is frequently easier than identifying the cause. Treatment should not be delayed until the diagnosis is available (Table 1.31).

Table 1.30: Postoperative causes of low cardiac output.

Reduced preload	Reduced contractility	Increased afterload
Hypovolaemia	Myocardial ischaemia and damage	Vasoconstriction
Cardiac tamponade	Arrhythmias	Fluid overload
Tension pneumothorax	Hypoxia	
Right ventricular dysfunction	Hypercapnia	
Positive pressure ventilation	Acidosis	

Table 1.31: Treatment of low cardiac output.

1	Ensure adequate oxygenation and ventilation
2	Consider and exclude cardiac tamponade
3	Optimise preload
4	Optimise heart rate and rhythm
5	Assess and improve myocardial contractility
6	Manipulate afterload

Specific complications

- Cardiac tamponade: should be considered and excluded in the presence of low cardiac output with elevated filling pressure and active mediastinal bleeding (particularly following active bleeding that has suddenly stopped). Equilibration of intracardiac pressures with RA = PAOP = LA, widening of the mediastinum on CXR, tachycardia, decreased ECG voltage help confirm the diagnosis. Untreated, tamponade results in PEA. Treatment is urgent surgical exploration.

- Cardiac herniation: rare complication of intrapericardial pneumonectomy resulting from the heart becoming displaced or entrapped in a pericardial defect. Treatment is immediate re-operation.

Respiratory
Atelectasis

Is commonest and occurs due to:

- Airway occlusion by mucous plugging of small airways.
- Bronchospasm.
- Shallow breathing due to pain.
- Compression of the lung by pneumothoraces, haemothoraces and intra-operative handling.

Atelectasis increases the work of breathing, impairs gas exchange and predisposes to pneumonia.

Pneumonia

Diagnosis is confirmed by hypoxia, tachypnoea and fever in addition to bronchial breathing on auscultation and consolidation on CXR. Treatment is aimed at clearing the airways and expanding the lung. Adequate analgesia and good physiotherapy form the basis of prevention and treatment. Nasotracheal aspiration, bronchoscopy and minitracheostomy may be indicated for patients with copious secretions.

Cardiogenic pulmonary oedema

May occur due to ventricular dysfunction and associated elevated pulmonary artery pressure. After pulmonary resection, atrial arrhythmias can lead to respiratory compromise particularly in the patient with limited respiratory reserve:

- Non-cardiogenic pulmonary oedema: associated with inappropriate fluid retention. Pulmonary endothelial damage arising from complement activation secondary to the inflammatory response to CPB, blood products or intra-operative lung trauma may result in interstitial pulmonary oedema.

- Haemodilution: associated with the initiation of CPB may lead to pulmonary oedema due to a reduction in oncotic pressure.

Pleural spaces, pneumothorax, pleural effusion

Persistence of a pleural space postoperatively is associated with complications because of the potential for fluid and air accumulation, which may result in the development of a pneumothorax, haemothorax or pleural effusion. Following lung resection the pleural space is normally obliterated by expansion of the remaining lung tissue, mediastinal deviation, diaphragmatic elevation and collapse of the intercostal spaces.

Tension pneumothorax

The presence of an intrathoracic drain does not exclude this. The drain may become blocked or kinked (particularly if placed posterior to the mid-axillary line). A tension pneumothorax may also occur in the contralateral lung. In the presence of unexpected low cardiac output, particularly in a ventilated patient, the diagnosis should always be considered.

Chylothorax

The thoracic duct may be damaged during mobilisation of the oesophagus before resection or anti-reflux procedures. Continued daily drainage of large volumes of serosanguineous fluid (> 800 ml/24 h) from the chest drains suggests the diagnosis. Management is initially conservative with chest drainage and a low elemental diet. Failure of non-operative management prompts re-operation and ligation of the duct.

Diaphragmatic dysfunction

Occurs following trauma to the phrenic nerve either by direct injury, devascularisation, retraction or topical ice used during cardiac procedures.

Lobar torsion

Rare complication following pulmonary resection or thoracic trauma resulting in the lobe rotating on its bronchovascular pedicle. It most commonly affects the right middle lobe following right upper lobectomy but also has been reported in other lobes. Diagnosis is by CXR and bronchoscopy. Treatment is immediate re-operation to prevent infarction.

Renal
Postoperative renal dysfunction

The principal aetiology of postoperative renal dysfunction is low cardiac output. Postoperative renal dysfunction falls into three categories:

- Transient rise in serum creatinine that resolves without the need for renal supportive therapy.

- Prolonged episode of renal dysfunction requiring temporary support with haemofiltration or haemodialysis but renal function recovers.

- Permanent renal failure.

Post-cardiac surgery oliguric renal failure requiring dialysis is associated with a 50% mortality rate.

Urinary retention

The majority of patients are catheterised but if not urinary retention is a common postoperative complication and is particularly associated with the use of epidural analgesia.

Gastrointestinal
Haemorrhage

GI haemorrhage may occur due to gastritis, duodenitis or peptic ulceration (particularly following systemic heparinisation required for CPB).

Intrathoracic or intra-abdominal bleeding may occur following mobilisation of the oesophagus or stomach. Division of the short gastric arteries before gastric mobilisation can result in trauma to the spleen, which if unrecognised may lead to significant postoperative bleeding or delayed splenic rupture.

Other complications of oesophageal surgery

- Anastomotic leak/perforation.

- Vagal nerve injury.

- Conduit ischaemia.

- Stricture formation.

- Delayed gastric emptying.

- Functional abnormalities.

- Hiatal hernia.

- Acalculous and calculous cholecystitis.

- Pancreatitis.

- Mesenteric ischaemia.

- Paralytic ilcus.

Neurological
Peripheral nerve injury

Traction to the brachial plexus can occur during sternotomy resulting in a temporary weakness or paraesthesia principally affecting the ulnar nerve that usually
resolves over several months. Avoidance is preferable to treatment.

Central nervous system injury

Spectrum of outcomes, from coma through specific motor deficits and confusion
to neuropsychological or cognitive impairment which may be temporary or permanent. More commonly associated with cardiac surgery and the use of CPB.

Cross-reference
Chapter 36, p. 347. CSiG

2

RESPIRATORY

MECHANICS AND CONTROL OF RESPIRATION

Definitions

- Ventilation is the movement of air from the atmosphere to the alveoli during inspiration, and in the reverse direction during expiration.

- Respiration is the act of gaseous exchange between:

  - oxygen, diffusing from the lung into the capillary network.

  - carbon dioxide, diffusing out of the bloodstream into the alveolus.

Physiology

Inspiration is an active process, initiated by inspiratory neurones in the respiratory centre, located in the floor of the fourth ventricle in the brainstem. To initiate a breath the respiratory centre stimulates the respiratory muscles via the cranial and spinal nerves.

- The diaphragm is the principal muscle of respiration, accounting for ~75% of the volume change.

  - as it contracts, it flattens, displacing the abdominal contents forward and downward.

  - ↑ intrathoracic volume → ↓ intrathoracic pressure (subatmospheric).

  - transpulmonary pressure difference between atmospheric at the lips and the negative pressure in the alveoli drives the air into the lungs during inspiration.

- Accessory muscles of respiration are responsible for preventing the collapse of the airways caused by the negative intrathoracic pressure during inspiration.

  - intercostal muscles contract to stabilise the chest wall, and contribute to the 'bucket handle' outer expansion of the lower ribs, which further increases intrathoracic volume.

  - dilator muscles of the upper airway contract, maintaining patency during inspiration.

The lungs and chest wall contain stretch and mechanoreceptors, which signal the inspiratory centre via the vagus nerve to end inspiration. The stretch receptors are also responsible for the Hering–Breuer reflex, which inhibits further inspiration when the lung is already inflated.

Expiration is a passive process of elastic recoil:

- Facilitated by the stored energy of the expanded chest wall following inspiration.

- Inspiratory neurones in the brainstem then start firing in response to afferent input from the stretch receptors on expiration.

Air is moved by convection from the lips to the terminal bronchioles and then by diffusion across the alveoli into the capillary network. Automatic respiration is controlled by the brainstem: the primary influences on its activity are from chemoreceptor feedback.

Control of respiration

- Central chemoreceptors lie close to the floor of the fourth ventricle and are intimately associated with the respiratory centre.

  - receptors are sensitive to changes in the pH of the interstitial fluid that surrounds them.

  - hydrogen (H^+) and bicarbonate (HCO_3^-) diffuse slowly between blood and the cerebospinal fluid (CSF), but CO_2 moves freely, allowing rapid reflection of blood CO_2 in the CSF.

  - $\uparrow CO_2 \rightarrow \downarrow\downarrow$ pH (since the CSF has little buffering capacity).

  - pH change is detected by the central chemoreceptors and stimulates the respiratory centre to increase minute volume.

  - CO_2 change in CSF is eventually buffered by the slower diffusion of HCO_3^- across the blood–brain barrier.

- Peripheral chemoreceptors in the aorta and carotid bodies are sensitive to the PaO_2 of arterial blood and start discharging once $PaO_2 < 13$ kPa (in healthy adults), causing an increase in the minute ventilation.

  - CO_2 homeostasis is usually the predominant influence on the control of ventilation.

  - role of O_2 becomes important during acute hypoxia, e.g. chest infection or patients with CO_2 retention, e.g. chronic bronchitis, who may rely on hypoxic drive. This, however represents only the minority of patients with COAD.

  - effects of hypercarbia and hypoxia summate in increasing minute volume.

The cerebral cortex is able to exert voluntary control over brainstem automatic ventilation. This can be modified by:

- Speech, eating, drinking and sleeping.

- Sneezing, yawning and vomiting.

- Activity and anticipation of exercise.

- Fever and hypothermia.

Lung volumes

These can be derived by spirometry and vary depending on age, sex, and size (height being a closer correlate than weight) (Figure 2.1).

Definitions

- Total lung capacity (TLC = 6 litres): volume of air in the lungs at the end of a maximal inspiration:

  $$TLC = IRV + ERV + V_t + RV$$
  $$= VC + RV.$$

- Tidal volume (V_t = 0.5 litres): volume of air inspired and expired during quiet breathing.

- Inspiratory reserve volume (IRV = 3.3 litres): maximal volume of air that can be inspired above tidal (V_t) inspiration.

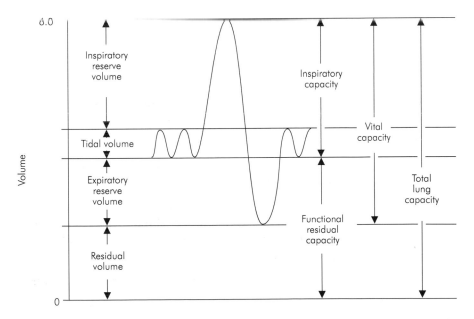

Figure 2.1: Spirometer trace of lung volumes (Reproduced from Fundamentals of Anaesthesia, GMM 1999).

- Expiratory reserve volume (ERV = 1 litre): maximal volume of air that can be expelled after tidal (V_t) expiration.

- Vital capacity (VC = 4.8 litres): maximal volume of air that can be expired following a maximal inspiration, i.e. V_t + IRV + ERV.

- Residual volume (RV = 1.2 litres): volume of air remaining in the lung after a maximal expiration.

- Functional residual capacity (FRC = 2.2 litres): volume of air remaining in the lung after tidal (V_t) expiration. This volume of air continues to take part in gaseous exchange at the end of expiration and allows a method for continuous oxygenation throughout the respiratory cycle. Its importance, therefore, is as an oxygen reserve.

- Closing capacity (CC): lung volume where small airways begin to collapse on expiration. Normally CC ≤ FRC. If CC ≥ FRC, then there will be airway closure, leading to collapse during tidal (quiet) ventilation, resulting in arterial hypoxaemia. Thus, any factor that decreases FRC will increase the risk of airway closure and collapse.

The factors affecting FRC are given in Table 2.1.

Table 2.1: Factors affecting FRC.

Factors increasing FRC	Factors decreasing FRC
PEEP/CPAP	extremes of age (very young and old)
Obstructive airways disease, e.g. asthma, emphysema	supine posture
	anaesthesia
	obesity
	abdominal/thoracic surgery*
	pulmonary disease, e.g. oedema or fibrosis

*Effects of surgery on lung volume can last for up to 2 weeks, causing: ↓ VC by 45% and ↓ FRC by 25%. These effects are seen most significantly in upper abdominal and thoracic operations.

Respiratory compliance

Compliance = change in volume (litres)/change in pressure (kPa).

This is defined as the change in lung volume brought about per unit charge in intrapleural pressure.

This measurement gives an indication of distensiability of the lungs, and therefore the amount of work needed to expand them during inspiration. Compliance curves form a characteristic sigmoid shape with increasing pressure (Figure 2.2). The slope of the line gives the measure of compliance. The steeper the slope of this line the greater the compliance, so less pressure is required to produce a unit rise in volume or alternatively more volume can be inspired per unit change in pressure.

Factors decreasing compliance:

- Extremes of lung volume (at low lung volumes there is collapse of small airways and alveoli and at high lung volumes the elastic fibres of the lung are fully stretched and large pressures are required to further increase volume).

- Extremes of age.

- Supine posture.

- Pregnancy (because of diaphragmatic splinting).

- ARDS.

- Pulmonary oedema/fibrosis.

- Ankylosing spondylitis.

- Kyphoscoliosis.

Ventilation of patients with decreased lung compliance leads to large increases in airway pressure per unit change in volume. This risks barotrauma, damaging the lungs and further reducing the compliance.

Dynamic compliance is measured during gas flow and forms a characteristic loop

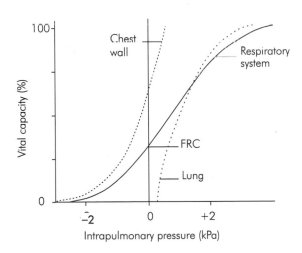

Figure 2.2: Lung and chest wall compliance (Reproduced from Fundamentals of Anaesthesia, GMM 1999).

(Figure 2.3). This is caused by the increased effort needed during inspiration to overcome the elastic forces resisting lung expansion. Normal expiration is a passive process driven by the stored energy from inspiration. The difference between the curves is termed hysteresis

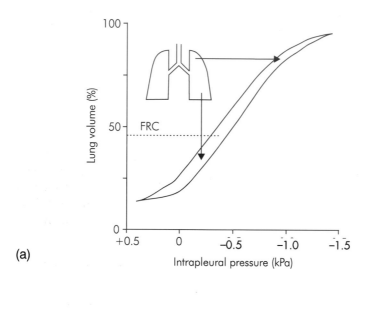

(a)

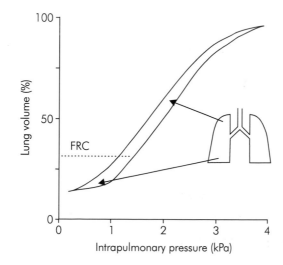

(b)

Figure 2.3: (a) Compliance during spontaneous ventilation. (b) Compliance during mechanical ventilation.

Ventilation and perfusion

Distribution of ventilation is uneven during inspiration. During spontaneous respiration, the majority of inspired gas passes to the lower (dependent) parts of the lung. This is because there is more negative pressure generated at the base than at the apex, favouring greater expansion. Blood flow is also greater at the base of the lung, owing to the increased hydrostatic pressure. Thus, during spontaneous respiration there is good matching of ventilation (V) and perfusion (Q). Matching of ventilation to perfusion prevents the development of hypoxaemia, which may result from:

- Shunt: perfused areas with inadequate ventilation.

- Dead-space: ventilated areas with inadequate perfusion.

The situation is reversed during mechanical (positive pressure) ventilation where preferential ventilation tends towards the upper (non-dependent) areas of the lung. This decreases the dependent lung volume and increases V/Q mismatch, leading to arterial hypoxaemia. The lung has a mechanism whereby it can improve matching of V/Q by diverting blood away from areas with poor ventilation. This is termed hypoxic pulmonary vasoconstriction (HPV) and results in decreasing the amount of shunted blood, thereby improving arterial hypoxaemia:

- Hypoxaemia that occurs as a result of shunt cannot be improved by increasing the oxygen concentration.

- General anaesthetics obliterate HPV and this is one reason why supplemental oxygen is required in patients during and after anaesthesia.

INTERPRETATION OF SPECIAL INVESTIGATIONS

Pulmonary function tests

These tests of dynamic lung performance are used to assess forced expiration, and are measured with a spirometer.

Uses

- Aid diagnosis.
- Quantify pulmonary impairment.
- Monitor the disease process.
- Monitor the response to therapy.

Forced expiration

- FVC (forced vital capacity): the volume is often less than that achieved by measurement from slow expiration.

- FEV_1 (forced expiratory volume): volume of the vital capacity breath expired in the first second.

The FEV_1/FVC ratio can be used to help distinguish obstructive from restrictive limitation to expired airflow. Normally, $FEV_1/FVC = 0.8$ (Figure 2.4).

- In restrictive conditions both the FEV_1 and FVC are reduced, but the ratio is typically normal or increased, e.g. pulmonary conditions such as fibrosis or chest wall restrictions such as kyphoscoliosis or flail chest.

- In obstructive conditions, FEV_1 is reduced to a far greater degree than the FVC; hence, the ratio is much lower, e.g. for asthma and emphysema (Table 2.2).

Table 2.2: FEV_1/FVC ratio.

	FEV_1	FVC	Ratio
Restrictive	↓↓	↓↓	normal or ↑
Obstructive	↓↓↓	↓	↓

Peak expiratory flow rate (PEFR)

This is used in obstructive airway conditions to assess treatment effects and reversibility. It is measured with a peak flow meter (the best of at least three attempts is the value recorded).

PEFR is reduced with:

- Asthma.
- COPD.
- Upper airway obstruction.
- Tracheal stenosis.
- Poor expiratory effort, e.g. musculoskeletal problems affecting the chest wall.

Arterial blood gases

Normal values:

- pH: 7.35–7.45.
- PCO_2: 4.4–5.8 kPa (33–44 mmHg).
- PO_2: 10.0–13.3 kPa (75–100 mmHg).

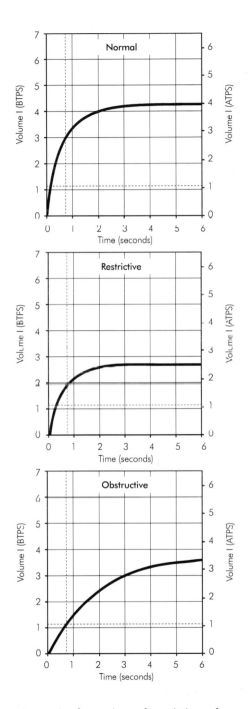

Figure 2.4 Spirometric tests in obstructive and restrictive pulmonary disease (Reproduced from Fundamentals in Anaesthesia, GMM 1999).

- SBC/HCO$_3$: 20–30 mmol l^{-1}.
- ABE/SBE: –2.5 to 2.5 mmol l^{-1}.
- SAT: 95–98%.

Check individual departmental values for normal range.

Definition of terms used

- pH:
  - –ve logarithm (base$_{10}$) of the H$^+$ content in blood.
  - inversely proportional to blood H$^+$ concentration; therefore, as pH decreases, so H$^+$ concentration rises, e.g. (Table 2.3):

Table 2.3: Relationship between pH and H$^+$ concentration.

pH	H$^+$ concentration (nmol l^{-1})
7.0	100
7.2	63
7.4	40
7.6	25

- SBC (standard bicarbonate): measure of plasma bicarbonate corrected to a PCO$_2$ of 5.3 kPa, removing the influence of respiratory effects on pH.
- ABE (actual base excess): *in vitro* measurement of metabolic acidosis (+ve) or alkalosis (–ve). PCO$_2$ is corrected to 5.3 kPa.
- SBE (standard base excess): *in vivo* assessment of acid–base balance since it adjusts for the buffering of haemoglobin and plasma proteins in whole blood compared with interstitial fluid.

Temperature has a significant effect on the results of ABG analysis:

- Decreasing temperature decreases pH (normal pH at 27°C is 7.25).
- Decreasing temperature decreases PO$_2$.

Therefore:

- It is essential to key the correct body temperature into the blood gas analyser when processing samples.
- Samples should be analysed as soon as possible after they have been taken to improve the accuracy of the results.

Acid–base homeostasis

Maintenance of constant body pH is important for homeostasis and the functioning of all cells in the body. Deviations from normal pH lead to dysfunction of essential organ systems and if severe and prolonged can result in death. The maintenance of constant pH is a function of the body's buffer systems:

- Bicarbonate: accounts for two-thirds of the body's buffering capacity:

  $$H_2O + CO_2 \leftrightarrow H_2CO_3 \leftrightarrow H^+ + HCO_3^-.$$

  This is an open buffer system since the components can be varied independently of each other, i.e. CO_2 may be removed by the lungs and HCO_3^- removed by the kidneys.

- Haemoglobin (Hb) within the erythrocytes: deoxygenated Hb has greater buffering capacity than oxygenated Hb.

- Phosphate.

- Plasma proteins.

Acid–base disturbances

- Acidosis: pH < 7.35.

- Alkalosis: pH > 7.45.

- Primary change in $PaCO_2$ is respiratory.

- Primary change in HCO_3 is metabolic (non-respiratory).

These changes can either be:

- Uncompensated: pH deficit remains uncorrected.

- Partially compensated: pH is returned towards normal.

- Fully compensated: pH is returned to normal.

Metabolic acidosis ($\downarrow$ pH, $\downarrow$ HCO$_3^-$)

Causes

- Increased H^+ production:

  - ketoacidosis.

  - lactic acidosis, e.g. tissue hypoxia from shock.

  - drugs, e.g. ethanol, salicylates.

- Decreased H^+ excretion: renal failure.

- HCO_3^- loss:
  - diarrhoea.
  - enteric losses, e.g. pancreatic, intestinal or biliary fistulae.
- Acid ingestion.

Compensation

- ↓ PCO_2 by hyperventilation.
- ↓ H^+ by kidneys (if no renal failure).

Management

- Treat the underlying cause wherever possible.
- Use of $NaHCO_3$ infusions are for severe and unresponsive cases only, as this is a considerable Na^+ and CO_2 load that can worsen intracellular acidosis.
- It may be necessary to consider haemofiltration for refractory severe acidosis.

Examples

Case 1

Uncompensated ketoacidosis in young insulin-dependent diabetic:

pH: 7.1.

PCO_2: 2.8 kPa.

PO_2: 13.0 kPa.

HCO_3^-: 7 mmol l⁻¹.

SBC: 8 mmol l⁻¹.

ABE: –21 mmol l⁻¹.

SBE: –20 mmol l⁻¹.

Saturation: 96%.

Hb: 14.0 g dl⁻¹.

Glucose: 22 mmol l⁻¹.

Case 2

Uncompensated lactic acidosis associated with hypotension from blood loss after rupture of AAA in a 70-year-old. Note that the degree of respiratory compensation is less than in the first case since the ability of this patient to hyperventilate is decreased owing to age:

pH: 7.1.

PCO_2: 3.5 kPa.

PO_2: 10.0 kPa.

HCO_3^-: 8 mmol l^{-1}.

SBC: 9 mmol l^{-1}.

ABE: −18 mmol l^{-1}.

SBE: −16.5 mmol l^{-1}.

Saturation: 93%.

Hb: 9.0 g dl^{-1}.

Glucose: 8 mmol l^{-1}.

Metabolic alkalosis (↑pH, ↑ HCO_3^-)

Causes

- Loss of H^+:
  - renal, e.g. diuretic therapy, hypokalaemia, mineralocorticoid excess (Cushing's and Conn's syndromes).
  - GIT, e.g. vomiting (pyloric stenosis, aspiration).
- Ingestion of HCO_3^- (usually iatrogenic).

Compensation

- ↑ PCO_2 by hypoventilation (limited by hypoxia).
- ↓ HCO_3^- by kidneys (when possible).

Management

- Diagnosis and treatment of the precipitating cause.
- Specific therapy is not usually required.
- With documented hypochloraemia and hypovolaemia the use of normal saline may be indicated.

Example
Case 3

A patient known to have longstanding peptic ulcer disease with persistent vomiting secondary to pyloric stenosis. There is some respiratory compensation.

pH: 7.56.

PCO_2: 7.2 kPa.

PO_2: 10.0 kPa.

HCO_3–: 45 mmol l^{-1}.

SBC: 35 mmol l^{-1}.

ABE: 10 mmol l^{-1}.

SBE: 6 mmol l^{-1}.

Saturation: 92%.

Hb: 11.0 g dl^{-1}.

Respiratory acidosis (↓ pH, ↑ PCO_2)

This is usually caused by hypoventilation due to:

- Airway obstruction: asthma, COAD, aspiration.

- Central depression: drugs, trauma, tumours.

- Neuromuscular disease: polio, Guillain Barré, motor neurone disease.

- Pulmonary disease: pneumonia, ARDS, pulmonary fibrosis.

- Chest wall disease: trauma (flail chest), kyphoscoliosis.

Compensation

- ↑ HCO_3^- by bicarbonate buffer system.

- ↓ H^+ by kidneys (can take several days).

Management

- Improve or reverse the respiratory failure, which may require mechanical ventilation.

- Associated hypoxaemia secondary to hypoventilation is the major threat to life and must be reversed quickly.

- The respiratory acidosis may be acute or chronic (or acute on chronic).

Examples

Case 4

Uncompensated acute respiratory acidosis in a young trauma patient with a flail chest.

pH: 7.25.

PCO_2: 8 kPa.

PO_2: 8 kPa.

HCO_3-: 25 mmol l^{-1}.

SBC: 24 mmol l^{-1}.

ABE: 2 mmol l^{-1}.

SBE: 1.5 mmol l^{-1}.

Saturation: 90%.

Hb: 12.0 g dl^{-1}.

Case 5

An elderly patient known to have chronic airways obstruction, with an acute exacerbation due to pneumonia causing (Table 2.4):

(a) Respiratory acidosis.

(b) Patient's condition deteriorates.

(c) He needs a period of mechanical ventilation, improving the clinical picture.

(d) Ventilation returns the CO_2 towards normal but this is an overcorrection for this patient and he becomes alkalotic.

Table 2.4: Blood gases for case 5.

	(a)	(b)	(c)	(d)
pH	7.3	7.25	7.4	7.55
PCO_2 (kPa)	9.0	10.5	7.5	5.5
PO_2 (kPa)	7.8	7.0	10.0	10.0
HCO_3- (mmol l^{-1})	38	38	36	38
SBC (mmol l^{-1})	31	31	30	31
ABE (mmol l^{-1})	10	10	10	10
SBE (mmol l^{-1})	14	14	14	14
Saturation (%)	88	83	94	94
Hb (g dl^{-1})	16.0			

Respiratory alkalosis ($\uparrow$pH, $\downarrow$PCO$_2$)

This is usually caused by hyperventilation due to:

- Hypoxia: altitude, anaemia.

- Central stimulation

    - drugs, e.g. salicylates.

    - head injury or brain tumours.

    - sepsis.

- Pulmonary disease: pneumonia, pulmonary oedema or embolism.

- Iatrogenic: mechanical ventilation.

Compensation

- $\downarrow$ HCO$_3^-$ by bicarbonate buffer system.

- $\uparrow$ H$^+$ by kidneys (can take several days).

Examples

Case 6

Uncompensated acute respiratory alkalosis from postoperative pneumonia.

pH: 7.55.

PCO$_2$: 3.8 kPa.

PO$_2$: 6.5 kPa.

HCO$_3^-$: 25 mmol l^{-1}.

SBC: 24 mmol l^{-1}.

ABE: 2.0 mmol l^{-1}.

SBE: 1.5 mmol l^{-1}.

Saturation: 85%.

Hb: 10.0 g dl^{-1}.

Case 7

Salicylate overdose that shows a combined respiratory alkalosis and metabolic acidosis.

pH: 7.45.

PCO$_2$: 2.7 kPa.

PO$_2$: 13 kPa.

HCO$_3^-$: 15 mmol l^{-1}.

SBC: 18 mmol l^{-1}.

ABE: −9 mmol l^{-1}.

SBE: −9.5 mmol l^{-1}.

Saturation: 97%.

Hb: 11.0 g dl^{-1}.

Cross-reference

Chapter 37, p. 359. CSiG

Interpretation of the chest radiograph

- Is it the correct patient?
- Look for suspected pathology.
- Systematic review:
  - Trachea: deviation.
  - Lungs and pleura:
    - pleural space: haemothorax, pneumothorax.
    - Lungs: infiltrates (contusions), hila, costophrenic regions.
  - Mediastinum:
    - cardiac injury: heart size (normal CTR < 0.55).
    - vascular injury: aortic rupture (widened mediastinum).
  - Diaphragm: disruption: bowel gas/NG tube above diaphragm.
  - Bones:
    - clavicle.
    - scapula.
    - ribs.
    - sternum.
  - Soft tissues: air under the diaphragm (pneumoperitoneum).

- Tubes and lines:
    - ET tube.
    - chest tube.
    - central line.
    - nasogastric tube.
    - pacemaker.
    - ECG leads.
- Technical aspects:
    - Central: clavicles equidistant from spinous process.
    - Penetration: lower thoracic vertebra visible through the heart.

Further reading

Radiology Made Easy (London: Greenwich Medical Media).

HYPOXIA

Hypoxia is reduced oxygen delivery to the tissues of the body:

$$DO_2 = CO \times [(H \times {}^{Sat}/_{100} \times 1.34) + (PaO_2 \times 0.003)],$$

where:

- DO_2 is oxygen delivery.
- CO is cardiac output.
- $Hb \times {}^{Sat}/_{100} \times 1.34$ is amount of oxygen carried by haemoglobin in the blood (1.34 is a calculation constant).
- $PaO_2 \times 0.003$ is amount of oxygen dissolved in blood and is usually negligible compared with that combined to haemoglobin.

There are several types of hypoxia depending on where the reduction in oxygen delivery occurs.

Hypoxic hypoxia

This results in ↓ Sat and ↓ PaO_2 and is caused by:

- Low oxygen concentration of the inspired gas mixture, e.g. at altitude.
- Hypoventilation, e.g. atelectasis and airway collapse, airway obstruction, drugs (opioids and anaesthetic agents), central depression of ventilation.

- Diffusion failure between the alveolus and capillary, e.g. pulmonary oedema and fibrosis or pneumonia.

- Ventilation/perfusion imbalance, e.g. ARDS.

- Shunting of blood from the venous to arterial circulation, e.g. cyanotic heart disease.

Anaemic hypoxia

This is the result of low Hb, which may be caused by:

- ↓ RBC from ↓ production, blood loss or ↑ destruction.

- ↓ Hb per RBC, e.g. hypochromic anaemia of iron deficiency.

- Abnormal forms of Hb, e.g. sickle cell disease.

- Reduced binding of oxygen to Hb, e.g. carbon monoxide poisoning.

At rest anaemic hypoxia is not usually a problem, unless the patient has co-existing ischaemic heart disease. During exercise, there can be severe limitation.

Stagnant hypoxia

This is due to a low cardiac output and causes high oxygen extraction leading to lower venous oxygen content. There is also decreased removal of waste products of metabolism leading to the accumulation of lactate (metabolic acidosis).

Histotoxic hypoxia

Here the delivery of oxygen to the tissues is adequate but they are unable to utilise it, e.g. cyanide poisoning.

Oxygen therapy

Hypoxaemia can occur with any patient after surgery. Some groups of patients are at higher risk, and should receive prolonged oxygen therapy (at least 72 h):

- Ischaemic heart disease.

- Anaemia.

- Major abdominal (especially upper GIT) and thoracic operations.

- Hypotension/low CO (it is important to treat the cause).

- Hypothermia.

- Obese patients.

- Hyperthermia/sepsis.

- Shivering.

The latter three have an increased oxygen demand.

Oxygen delivery systems

Variable performance devices

The oxygen concentration delivered to the patient is not constant and depends on the minute volume (MV), or more specifically the peak inspiratory flow rate (PIFR). As PIFR increases, more air will be entrained from the surroundings and the oxygen concentration delivered to the patient will decrease, unless the oxygen flow rate is increased. Table 2.5 gives two examples of systems commonly used after surgery.

Table 2.5: Concentration of Oxygen delivered by Hudson mask and nasal specs.

Hudson mask O_2 flow (l min^{-1})	O_2 concentration (%)	Nasal specs O_2 flow (l min^{-1})	O_2 concentration (%)
2	24–38	1	25–29
4	35–45	2	29–35
6	51–61	4	32–39
8	57–67		
10	61–73		

Fixed-performance devices (Venturi masks)

These deliver a constant oxygen concentration independent of the patient's respiratory pattern (minute volume and PIFR). The oxygen supply entrains air at a fixed rate via a jet built into the mask. The total flow rate is, therefore, higher than the PIFR and dilution of the oxygen supply does not occur. The jet entrainment devices are colour-coded and higher flow rates must be dialled when increased oxygen concentrations are required (Table 2.6).

Table 2.6: Concentration of Oxygen delivered by Venturi masks.

Colour code	O_2 supply flow rate (l min^{-1})	Delivered O_2 concentration (%)
White	4	28
Yellow	8	35
Red	10	40
Green	15	60

Cross-reference

Falk van Rooyen I, Jones JG. Perioperative management of the adult patient with respiratory disease. *Surgery* 1999; 17: 97–101.   SURGERY

RESPIRATORY FAILURE

Respiratory failure occurs when the PO_2 and PCO_2 can no longer be maintained within normal limits. If untreated this leads on to cellular hypoxaemia and acidosis by decreasing the capacity for gaseous exchange. Respiratory failure may be split up into two types, depending on the carbon dioxide concentration present in blood. Patients may progress from one type to the other:

- Type I: ↓ PaO_2 with normal or ↓ $PaCO_2$ (there may be respiratory alkalosis):

  - pulmonary embolism.

  - fibrosing alveolitis.

  - pneumonia.

  - asthma.

  - early ARDS.

  - (the latter three conditions, when severe, are also associated with a type II failure.)

- Type II: ventilatory failure – ↓ PaO_2 with ↑ $PaCO_2$ (respiratory acidosis).

  - mechanical obstruction to the airway, e.g. vomit, blood, foreign body or tumour.

  - obstructive airways disease, e.g. COAD, severe asthma.

  - advanced ARDS.

  - severe pneumonia.

  - neuromuscular disorders, e.g. cervical cord injury, polio, Guillain Barré, motor neurone disease.

  - chest wall deformities, e.g. chest trauma (flail chest), ankylosing spondylitis, kyphoscoliosis.

  - central depression of respiratory drive, e.g. drugs (especially sedatives), head injury, brain tumours.

Signs of respiratory failure

- Tachypnoea.

- Dyspnoea.

- Tachycardia.

- Use of accessory muscles of respiration:

  - intercostal recession.

  - subcostal recession.

  - tracheal tug.

- Inability to speak in sentences (leading on to total inability to speak).

- Impaired consciousness (this is a grave sign).

- Cyanosis is a blue/purple discoloration of the skin caused by the presence of deoxyhaemoglobin (> 5 gdl⁻¹). This is a notoriously unreliable sign, particularly in areas with poor or artificial lighting. It is possible to observe:

  - cyanosis without hypoxia (polycythaemia).

  - hypoxia without cyanosis (anaemia).

RESPIRATORY SUPPORT: MECHANICAL VENTILATION

Positive pressure ventilation may be required for signs of respiratory failure (see previous section). The decision whether to institute ventilatory support should be taken by a senior clinician, and is based on several factors

- Premorbid health status of the patient is an important index of survivability following admission to the ICU.

- There should be potential reversibility of the admitting condition (see Chapter 5, ICU admission).

Indications for mechanical ventilation

- Inadequate ventilation:

  - apnoea.

  - RR > 35 min⁻¹ (normal range is 12–20 min⁻¹ for adults).

  - VC < 15 ml kg⁻¹ (normal range is 65–75 ml kg⁻¹).

  - Vt < 5 ml kg⁻¹ (normal range is 5–7 ml kg⁻¹).

  - $PaCO_2$ > 8 kPa (depends on the patient's normal $PaCO_2$).

- Inadequate oxygenation: PaO_2 < 8 kPa (breathing > 60% oxygen).

- Specific surgical indications:
  - Head injury
    - unprotected airway.
    - GCS < 8.
    - ↑ ICP.
  - Chest injury:
    - flail chest.
    - pulmonary contusion.
  - Facial trauma.
  - High spinal injury.

Intermittent positive pressure ventilation (IPPV)

The principle of IPPV is the same as for spontaneous ventilation. Gas flows down a pressure gradient from the mouth to the alveoli. The difference, however lies in that the proximal driving pressure is positive rather than atmospheric, and the distal pressure is zero rather than negative. Work is still done to expand the lung and chest wall and this is stored and used to drive expiration, which is passive. IPPV affects many body systems:

- Respiratory:
  - FRC is recovered, improving the efficiency of ventilation. The inspired oxygen concentration can be adjusted to optimise oxygenation, and carbon dioxide removal is improved in patients with respiratory failure.
  - lung water can be reduced, further improving oxygenation.
  - high pressures, sometimes needed to expand the lung, can cause damage due to barotrauma, leading to pneumothorax formation. This is especially true when the respiratory compliance is reduced, e.g. with ARDS. Subsequent ventilation with drained pneumothoraces can be difficult and inefficient, due to air leaks.
  - reduction of HPV, with resultant increased mismatching of ventilation and perfusion.
- Cardiovascular: overall ↓ in BP and CO:
  - ↑ preload (↓ venous return to the right ventricle) due to loss of negative pressure intrathoracic pump.

- ↓ pulmonary vascular resistance (PVR).
    - RV dilatation.
    - ↓ LV filling (because of volume increase in RV).
- sedation.
- correction of hypoxia, hypercarbia and acidosis decreases endogenous catecholamine drive on the CVS.
- Renal:
    - ↓ cardiac output results in:
        - ↓ renal blood flow.
        - ↓ renal perfusion pressure.
        - ↓ glomerular filtration rate.
        - ↓ urine output.
- Cerebral:
    - ↑ intrathoracic pressure →↑ ICP.
    - ↓ CO_2 →↓ cerebral blood volume →↓ ICP.
- Metabolic: titration of CO_2 levels to treat and correct acid–base disturbances.

Commencing mechanical ventilation

Once the appropriate patient has been selected (depending on the criteria previously mentioned) set the ventilator to deliver:

- $F_iO_2 = 0.5$.
- $V_t = 10{-}12$ ml kg^{-1}.
- RR = 10–12/h.
- I:E ratio = 1:2.
- Limit peak airway pressure (PAwP) to 40 cmH$_2$O.
- PEEP = 2.5–10 cmH$_2$O (where appropriate).

Regular arterial blood gases (ABG) should be taken following the initial mechanical ventilation of any patient. Some or all of the parameters may need to be changed depending on the individual needs of the patient.

Modes of ventilation

Controlled mandatory ventilation (CMV)

- Ventilator will deliver a set tidal volume (V_t) at a set respiratory rate (RR).

- Patient makes no inspiratory effort.

- Any attempt to breathe or cough by the patient during inspiration can result in dangerously high peak airway pressures (PAwP), leading to barotrauma.

- Patient must be deeply sedated and is often paralysed.

Synchronised intermittent mandatory ventilation (SIMV)

- Minute volume is composed of a mixture of mandatory V_t breaths (initiated by the ventilator) and some spontaneous breaths (initiated by the patient).

- Coordination (synchronisation) between the ventilator-initiated breaths and the patient-initiated breaths, so that both are not delivered simultaneously. This prevents the high PAwP sometimes seen with CMV.

- Patients may be less deeply sedated and muscle paralysis is rarely required.

SIMV has a number of advantages over CMV:

- ↓ level of sedation required.

- ↓ incidence of ↑ PAwP (hence, ↓ incidence of barotrauma).

- ↓ mean airway pressure (MA_wP) → less ↓ in CO and BP (greater haemodynamic stability).

- Better matching of ventilation and perfusion.

- Easier assessment of spontaneous breathing activity.

- Improved weaning from ventilation (less disuse atrophy of the respiratory muscles since spontaneous ventilation is not discouraged).

Pressure control ventilation (PCV)

CMV and SIMV are examples of volume controlled ventilation, where a preset volume is delivered to the patient. PCV differs in that the pressure is set and the volume delivered to the patient will vary depending on the compliance (see Mechanics & Control of Respiration) of the lungs and the inspiratory time:

- Patients with ↓ lung compliance will receive a ↓ V_t for any set pressure.

- Square wave pressure trace:

  - MA_wP is higher for any level of PAwP.

  - ↑ MA_wP equates with ↑ oxygenation.

- ↓ PAwP →↓ risk of barotrauma.

- RR set on ventilator.

- Start with pressure of 30 cmH$_2$O to give V_t = 10–12 ml kg^{-1} (depends on lung compliance).

Pressure support ventilation (PSV)

This is sometimes referred to as pressure assisted ventilation:

- Patient triggers the ventilator to deliver a preset pressure to the lungs.

- RR determined by the patient.

- V_t depends on the level of PS and the lung compliance.

- Set level of PS to give V_t = 10–12 ml kg^{-1} (usually 15–30 cmH$_2$O).

This mode of ventilation can be used in isolation or in conjunction with PCV or SIMV. Its main use is for weaning from ventilation, with the level of PS reduced as the mechanics of respiration improve:

- Minimal sedation needed (only to tolerate the ETT).

- Has the advantage of maintaining muscular activity, thereby minimising the risks of disuse atrophy.

For a summary of the different modes of ventilation, see Table 2.6.

Mechanisms to optimise lung volume

These manoeuvres increase FRC by alveolar recruitment, re-expanding collapsed areas of the lung. This places the lung on a more efficient (steeper) part of the compliance curve (see Mechanics & Control of Respiration), generating maximum volume change per unit increase in pressure. This improves oxygenation for any given F$_i$O$_2$:

- Continuous positive airways pressure (CPAP) is used during spontaneous ventilation.

- Positive end expiratory pressure (PEEP) is used during ventilator delivered breaths.

Table 2.6: Comparison of the different modes of mechanical ventilation.

	Tidal volume (V$_t$)	Respiratory rate (RR)	Peak airway pressure (PAwP)	Sedation requirement	Weaning mode	Use
CMV	set on ventilator	Set on ventilator	Dependent on pulmonary compliance	Yes	No	Standard post-operative ventilation mode
PCV	depends on pulmonary compliance	Set on ventilator	Limited/set on ventilator	Significant (may also require paralysis)	No	Ventilating uncompliant lungs e.g. ARDS
SIMV	mandatory breaths set on ventilator Spontaneous breaths determined by patient	Minimum rate set on ventilator Maximum rate determined by patient	Dependent on pulmonary compliance	Minimal/none	Yes	Initial weaning mode
PSV	dependent on pulmonary compliance	Determined by patient	Limited/set on ventilator	Minimal/none	Yes	Advanced weaning mode

- Inverse ratio ventilation (IRV). The usual I:E ratio of 1:2 gives adequate time for expiration, which is passive. Reversing the ratio to 1:1, 2:1 or 3:1 will progressively decrease the time for expiration, which will generate autoPEEP. This will ↑ MA$_w$P (without ↑↑ PAwP), thus improving oxygenation. This requires deep sedation and paralysis since this is a very unnatural and uncomfortable mode of ventilation.

Associated effects of these manoeuvres:

- ↑ Intrathoracic pressure →↓ venous return →↓ CO and BP.

- ↓ CO_2 elimination → respiratory acidosis.

Weaning from mechanical ventilation

This is re-instituting independent spontaneous respiration after a period of ventilatory support. The withdrawal of artificial ventilation is achieved gradually and success depends on several factors:

- Duration of mechanical ventilation: quicker weaning with postoperative cases (< 24 h ventilated).

- Past medical history: particularly respiratory and cardiovascular disease.

- Current medical problems: active chest infection, significant areas of collapse or consolidation, and heart failure greatly decrease the chances of success. These are relative contraindications to active weaning.

- Nutritional state and muscle power: this depends on many factors (see Chapter 3 Nutrition in the Critically Ill).

- Drugs: residual levels of opioids, sedatives and muscle relaxants will determine the effectiveness and speed of the weaning process.

Signs of failure during weaning

- Tachypnoea and dyspnoea.

- Hypoxia and hypercarbia.

- Use of accessory muscles of respiration (see Mechanics and Control of Respiration).

- Exhaustion leading to ↓ conscious level.

Weaning preconditions

- Starts only after recovery from the pathology that required ventilatory support.

- Haemodynamic stability.

- Optimisation of oxygen delivery to the tissues: Hb and Cardiac Output.

- Optimisation of nutritional status to prevent muscle fatigue.

- Active sepsis and pyrexia should be excluded since these increase oxygen demand and may lead to early failure.

- F_iO_2 should be < 0.6.

Practical aspects of weaning from ventilatory support

- Weaning plan should be started as early as possible in the day: ideally after the morning ward round.

- Minimise sedation and opioid analgesia: however bear in mind that pain ↑ O_2 demand →↑ risk of failure.

- Decrease mandatory respiratory rate delivered by the ventilator: gradually towards zero.

- Decrease the pressure support level: maintaining adequate V_t.

- Decrease PEEP.

- When:

  - SIMV rate = 0.

  - PS = 10 cmH$_2$O.

  - PEEP = 5 cmH$_2$O.

Then the patient may be put on a T-piece (± CPAP = 5 cmH$_2$O) for a few hours at a time, alternating with PS via the ventilator. Good clinical and ABG monitoring is required until the patient is able to maintain adequate ventilation independently. This process may take weeks to complete. There is currently no reliable predictor of successful weaning.

Cross-reference

Chapter 37, p. 363. CSiG

AIRWAY MANAGEMENT

Airway obstruction usually occurs in the unconscious patient and may be partial or complete. It may occur anywhere from the nose or mouth down to the trachea. There are many causes of an obstructed airway:

- Relaxation of the soft tissues (especially the tongue) in the oropharynx.

- Vomit, blood or other foreign body.

- Laryngospasm.

- Facial trauma.

- Oedema of the airway secondary to burns or smoke inhalation, infection or inflammation, and anaphylactoid reactions.

- Lower airway obstruction (sublaryngeal) is less common and associated with:

  - pulmonary secretions and mucous plugging (common in ICU patients).

  - thoracic trauma.

  - obstructive airways: asthma or emphysema (expiration).

  - pulmonary oedema.

  - large pneumothorax/haemothorax.

Clinical

- Complete obstruction is silent.

- Partial obstruction is noisy.

- There may be paradoxical (see-saw) movements of the chest and abdomen.

Manoeuvres designed to keep the airway patent aim to achieve the 'sniffing the morning air' position with the neck flexed and head extended:

- Head tilt: avoid in trauma patients.

- Chin lift.

- Jaw thrust: this is the safest method for patients with suspected neck injury (in conjunction with in-line stabilisation).

These techniques may be supplemented by:

- Oropharyngeal (Guedel) airway.

- Nasopharyngeal airway (not with suspected base-of-skull fracture).

- Laryngeal mask airway (LMA): is relatively easy to insert and rests in the hypopharynx cushioned by an air-filled cuff (Figure 2.5). Although not a definitive airway, this can be used for positive pressure ventilation (with a variable leak around the cuff).

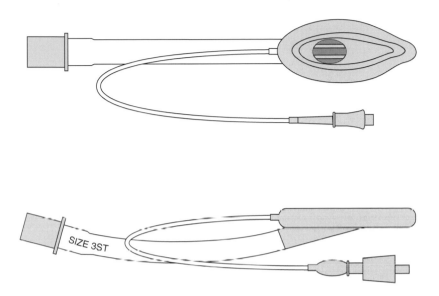

Figure 2.5: Laryngeal mask airway.

Definitive airway

- Endotracheal tube (ETT):
    - nasal is more comfortable and, therefore, requires less sedation.
    - oral makes suctioning and fibreoptic examination of the lower airway easier.
- Tracheostomy:
    - mini-tracheostomy.
    - percutaneous.
    - surgical.

Indications for a definitive airway

- Protection of the lower airway from aspiration by food, blood, secretions or vomit (any patient with a GCS < 8 will need airway protection).
- Facilitation of positive pressure ventilation.
- By-passing any upper airway obstruction.
- Allows regular suction of the lower airway and aspiration of samples for culture.

Principles of tracheal intubation

- Size of ETT.

    - calculate the correct size (internal diameter) for a child by: (age/4) + 4.

    - calculate the correct length (oral) for a child by: (age/12) + 12 cm.

    - approximate size for adult male oral ETT is 9.0 mm (internal diameter) cut to 23 cm (length).

    - approximate size for adult female oral ETT is 8.0 mm (internal diameter) cut to 21 cm (length).

- Unless the patient is deeply unconscious sedative drugs and muscle relaxants will be required to prevent sympathetic stimulation and coughing.

- Trained help should be available.

- Full monitoring and resuscitation drugs should be instantly available.

- Patient should be on a trolley or bed with the facility of tilting head down.

- Patient should be pre-oxygenated with 100% oxygen until SaO_2 = 100% (or as high as possible).

- Suction apparatus should be switched on and placed under the patient's pillow.

- Cricoid pressure (to occlude the oesophagus) is needed for tracheal intubation in patients with a suspected full stomach.

- Aides for difficult intubation (bougies) and other airway adjuncts should be available.

- A means to deliver positive pressure ventilation.

Bag ventilation

- Self-inflating bag:

    - connects to facemask, LMA, ETT or tracheostomy tube.

    - one-way valve to divert expired (waste) gas to the atmosphere.

    - self-inflates with air: unless an oxygen supply is attached:

        - 5–6 l min^{-1} gives F_iO_2 = ~0.45.

        - 10–15 l min^{-1} via a reservoir bag gives F_iO_2 = ~0.9.

- Rebreathing (anaesthetic) circuit:

  - connects to facemask, LMA, ETT or tracheostomy tube.

  - adjustable pressure limiting (APL) valve: used to vent the expired gas to the atmosphere. This keeps the bag inflated but can lead to ↑ CO_2 levels (hence, the term 'rebreathe').

  - APL valve can be used to provide PEEP.

  - more difficult to use than self inflating bag.

  - advantage is better visualisation and feel of the patient's spontaneous breathing pattern and effort.

Cross-reference

Trotter C, Noble DW. Management of the airway and acute airway obstruction. *Surgery* 1998; 16: 1–4.

ARDS

Acute respiratory distress syndrome (ARDS) is the pulmonary component of the systemic inflammatory response syndrome (SIRS) see p112.

Direct (pulmonary) causes

- Contusion from blunt trauma.
- Aspiration of stomach contents.
- Near drowning.
- Infection.
- Smoke or toxic inhalation.

Indirect (extrapulmonary) causes

- Sepsis.
- Major trauma.
- Embolic episodes (thrombotic, fat or amniotic).
- Pancreatitis.
- Massive blood transfusion.
- Severe or prolonged haemorrhage/hypotension.
- Disseminated Intravascular Coagulopathy (DIC).
- Cardiopulmonary bypass.

The incidence varies from 3 to 6 per 10^5 in the UK, up to 80 per 10^5 of the population in the USA. This variability has much to do with differences in diagnosis between the two countries, which led to a consensus conference formulating the following criteria:

- There must be a known precipitating cause.

- The onset of symptoms must be acute.

- There must be hypoxia refractory to oxygen therapy.

- There must be new bilateral, fluffy infiltrates on the CXR (this sign may lag behind the clinical picture by 12–24 h).

- There must be no cardiac failure or fluid overload (this is to exclude these causes of the typical CXR appearance in ARDS, and is taken as PAwP < 18 mmHg).

The severity of the hypoxic insult can be quantified into acute lung injury (ALI) or ARDS depending on the fraction of inspired oxygen that the subject is breathing:

- In ALI the PaO_2:F_iO_2 ratio is < 40 kPa (300 mmHg).

- In ARDS the PaO_2:F_iO_2 ratio is < 27 kPa (200 mmHg).

The following are associated clinical findings (but are not included as diagnostic criteria):

- Need for mechanical ventilation.

- Low lung compliance (see Mechanics & Control of Respiration).

- High airway pressures during positive pressure ventilation.

Pathophysiology

Early stages (within 24 h of the precipitating event) are shown in Figure 2.6.

The late stages are shown in Figure 2.7.

The disease process is not uniform within the lung, with some areas being spared and capable of gas exchange.

Clinical

This depends largely on the severity and extent of lung injury present. Spontaneously breathing patients are typically:

- Tachypnoeic.

- Dyspnoeic.

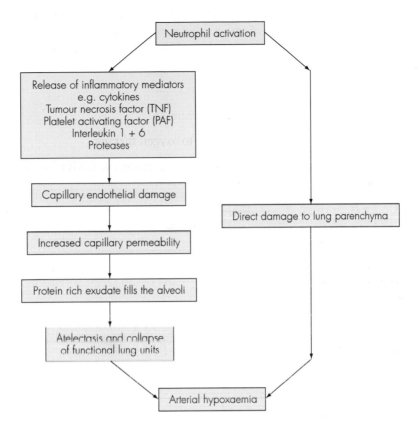

Figure 2.6: Early stages of ARDS.

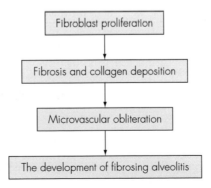

Figure 2.7: Late stages of ARDS.

- Exhibit a laboured breathing pattern often involving the accessory muscles of respiration.

- Presence of cyanosis is variable and depends largely on the level of deoxygenated haemoglobin present.

Management

- Identify and treat the underlying cause.

- Prevention of MOF by adequate fluid resuscitation with the judicious use of fluids to optimise haemodynamic stability without precipitant rises in PAwP, which may increase lung water and worsen hypoxia. This may require the use of a PAFC and inotropes.

- Respiratory support, where the aim is to achieve reasonable levels of oxygenation and carbon dioxide removal without any further damage to the lungs:

  - permissible hypercapnia to $PaCO_2$ of 10–15 kPa (if no signs of acidosis or cerebral oedema).

  - acceptable hypoxaemia to PaO_2 of 8 kPa (if no signs of ischaemia).

Methods of ventilatory support

Collapsed areas of the lung may be expanded by alveolar recruitment manoeuvres designed to increase the FRC, thereby improving oxygenation:

- CPAP (5–10 cmH_2O) can be used in spontaneously breathing patients in the early stages of the disease, and may be administered via a nasal or facemask. It is seldom effective for long-term therapy and is usually a holding measure.

- PEEP (10–15 cmH_2O) can be used during mechanical ventilation but is associated with haemodynamic instability.

Conventional volume controlled ventilation with tidal volumes of 10–12 ml kg^{-1} can cause barotrauma and volutrauma to the healthy areas of the lung. These can be avoided by the following manoeuvres:

- Use of pressure controlled ventilation: generates a characteristic square waveform so optimising mean airway pressure (MA_wP) without increasing peak airway pressure (PA_wP). The upper pressure is limited to that set on the ventilator. This is usually set to 30–40 cmH_2O.

- Use of inverse ratio ventilation: normal inspiratory (I):expiratory (E) ratio = 1:2, but this can lead to high inflation pressures because of the relatively short inspiratory time and the stiff lungs. I:E ratio may be prolonged to 1:1, 2:1 or 3:1. This will further optimise MA_wP, so improving oxygenation for any given PA_wP. There are several problems associated with these methods of ventilation:

- haemodynamic instability.

- decrease in carbon dioxide elimination leading to further hypercapnoea.

- deep sedation and paralysis are required since this is a very unnatural and uncomfortable mode of ventilation.

Resistant hypoxaemia may benefit from improved matching of ventilation (V) and perfusion (Q) by:

- Changing the position of the patient:

  - prone ventilation (usually for 4–8 h at a time). This strategy aims to decrease the collapse seen in the dependent areas of the lung by reducing the time that the patient spends in one position. Gradually the dependent areas in the new position will collapse and contribute towards hypoxaemia, and the position will need to be changed again. This can be very labour intensive for the nursing staff.

  - ventilation on a rotating bed. By continuously moving the patient through 90° areas of the lung will only become dependent transiently and, therefore, reduce the incidence of collapse.

  - both these manoeuvres are made more hazardous by the use of multiple infusion lines or haemofiltration.

- Prostacyclin and nitric oxide (NO), also known as endothelium-derived relaxant factor (EDRF). When delivered via a nebuliser, these agents selectively vasodilate the pulmonary vascular beds that are adequately ventilated, thus improving V/Q matching and improving hypoxaemia.

Complications

- Ventilator acquired infection: frequent cultures of bronchial aspirate and blood should be taken. Close liaison with the microbiology department will aid the rational use of antimicrobial agents and guide the choice of blind therapy when indicated.

- Pneumothorax: these may be multiple and drainage is often needed until the patient is breathing spontaneously. CT guidance may be required to aid the drainage of loculated pneumothoraces, as blind drainage can be catastrophic in severe cases.

- Multi-organ failure (MOF) (see Chapter 3 page 112 Multisystem failure and systemic inflammatory response syndrome).

Prognosis

This is extremely variable and the mortality is increased by:

- Increasing age.

- Significant past medical history: especially renal or hepatic failure.

- Precipitating cause: sepsis has the highest mortality and polytrauma (provided the patient survives the initial event) has the lowest.

- Associated complications increase morbidity and can worsen mortality.

Early deaths are often related to the precipitating cause, late deaths are frequently associated with MOF. Many survivors have little or no residual problems; others will have a range of disability from a reduced exercise tolerance to symptoms and signs of fibrotic lung disease.

3

OTHER SYSTEMS AND MULTISYSTEM FAILURE

HEAD INJURY

Richard Downs

One million patients present annually to A&E departments in the UK with head injuries. Of these, 150 000 are admitted to hospital and 3000 are transferred to a neurosurgical centre. Sixty percent are adults, of which 70% are males, and 25% have a history of recent alcohol intake. All patients with severe head injuries should be referred for a neurosurgical opinion. The principal aim of treatment of patients with head injuries is to prevent secondary brain injury.

Classification

The ATLS® Classification of Head Injuries is a simple yet comprehensive system (Table 3.1).

Table 3.1: ATLS® Classification of Head Injuries. Modified from American College of Surgeons Committee on Trauma. *ATLS® Student Manual* (Chicago: American College of Surgeons, 1997) with permission.

Classification			
Mechanism	blunt penetrating		
Severity	mild moderate severe	GCS 13–15 GCS 9–12 GCS < 8	
Morphology	skull fracture	vault basilar	
	intracranial	focal	extradural (epidural) (Figure 3.2) subdural (Figure 3.1) intracerebral (Figure 3.3)
		diffuse	concussion diffuse axonal injury

Pathophysiology
Primary brain injury

- Accounts for 50% of brain injury deaths.

- Occurs on impact and can be diffuse or focal.

- Due to shearing forces, which cause tearing of axonal tracts.

- Often, little can be done in the way of treatment.

- May result in secondary complications, which can be prevented and treated.

Secondary brain injury

The additional insult imposed on brain tissue following the primary brain injury. It can be extracranial or intracranial.

Extracranial causes are due to:

- Hypoxia from airway obstruction, loss of respiratory drive or pulmonary complications.

- Hypotension due to shock from other injuries.

The injured brain loses its ability to regulate its own blood supply and becomes vulnerable to ischaemic damage when hypoxia or hypotension occur.

Intracranial causes are due to raised intracranial pressure (ICP) from haematoma formation such as extradural haematoma or cerebral oedema.

- Raised ICP jeopardises cerebral perfusion pressure (CPP) as:

  CPP = MAP – ICP.

- If ICP is allowed to continue to rise compensatory mechanisms become exhausted and 'coning' occurs with brainstem death.

Infection in the form of meningitis or cerebral abscess may occur several days after the injury.

Management

Resuscitation of the patient as per ATLS® principles

- **Airway:**
  - ensure a clear airway and administer 100% oxygen while protecting the cervical spine with manual in-line immobilisation as there is a high possibility of cervical fracture in head-injured patients.
  - airway may be cleared initially with a chin lift or jaw thrust followed by an oral (Guedel) airway. An endotracheal tube may be necessary (see indications for intubation in Table 3.4).

- **Breathing:**
  - ensure adequacy of breathing once a clear airway is established.
  - may require positive pressure ventilation with an ambubag or ventilator.
  - arterial blood gas analysis is used to determine adequacy of ventilation.
  - $PaCO_2 > 6$ kPa requires intubation and ventilation.

- Circulation:

  - maintain a blood pressure at or above normal for the patient's age.

  - unexplained hypotension may be due to haemorrhage or an associated spinal cord injury.

  - use of IV fluids and blood as necessary.

  - source of haemorrhage should be sought and treated.

Once the patient is stable, a further assessment can be carried out.

Assessment of the severity of head injury

Clinical assessment is with the Glasgow Coma Score (Table 3.2). This should be repeated frequently as it is not only the absolute value that is important, but also the trend, indicating deterioration, stability or improvement.

Table 3.2: Glasgow Coma Score (GCS).

	Motor (M)	Verbal (V)	Eyes (E)
1	Nil	Nil	Nil
2	Extensor response	Incomprehensible sounds	To pain
3	Abnormal flexion	Inappropriate words	To speech
4	Withdraws	Confused conversation	Spontaneous
5	Localises	Orientated	
6	Obeys		

GCS = M + V + E.

Appropriate radiological imaging can then be performed. In an ideal world, all head injury patients would have a CT scan.

Indications for a skull X-ray

- There was loss of consciousness or a period of amnesia.

- There are neurological symptoms or signs.

- There is cerebrospinal fluid or blood otorrhoea or rhinorrhoea.

- Scalp injury of a serious nature.

- Suspected penetrating injury with CT not readily available.

Proceed to a CT scan (Figures 3.1–3) if:

- There is deterioration in conscious level as assessed by the GCS or pupillary signs develop.

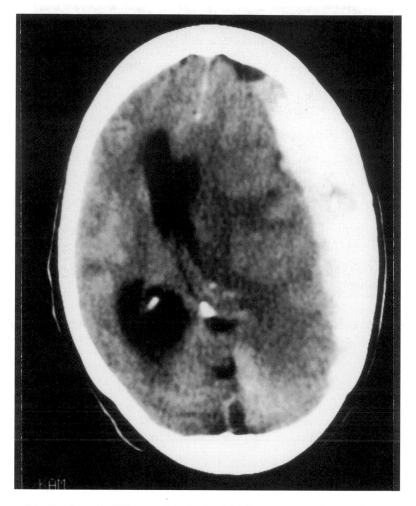

Figure 3.1: Section of a CT scan of the brain. A high attenuation abnormal area is in the subdural space on the left side. This is compressing the normal left cerebral hemisphere and is causing a mass effect such that there is compression of the left lateral ventricle and a shift of the midline to the right. These are the features of an acute subdural haematoma (Reproduced from Radiology Made Easy, GMM, 1999).

- There is development of focal neurological signs.

- There is a fractured skull.

- The patient remains confused or in a state of unconsciousness.

- The patient is difficult to assess, e.g. alcohol.

- There is a penetrating injury.

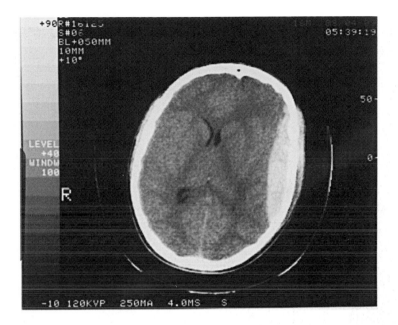

Figure 3.2: CT scan of a patient showing an extradural haematoma with a considerable shift of the midline (Reproduced from Textbook of Neuranaesthesia and Critical Care, GMM, 2000).

A neurosurgeon should be consulted if:

- There is a fractured skull with contusion or a decreased level of consciousness, seizures or any neurological symptoms or signs.

- There is persistence of coma (GCS < 8) despite adequate resuscitation.

- There is a deterioration in the level of consciousness (GCS ↓ 2).

- Confusion or other neurological disturbance persists for > 8 h.

- There is a compound depressed skull fracture or a suspected basal skull fracture.

- CT scan is abnormal.

- The patient is a child with a tense fontanelle.

The following groups of patients should be admitted to a critical care facility (Table 3.3).

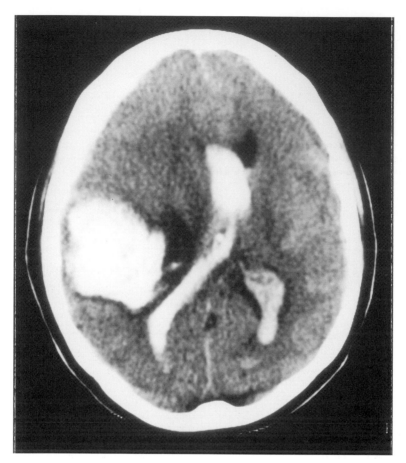

Figure 3.3: Section of a CT scan showing a very large right-sided intracerebral haematoma. The blood is fresh because the attenuation is white. Fresh bleeding causes a mass effect with a midline shift to the left side, away from the lesion. In addition there is a high attenuation (white) area in the lateral ventricles. This is due to there being an intraventricular haemorrhage (Reproduced from Radiology Made Easy, GMM, 1999).

Table 3.3: Indications for critical care admission for head injury.

Intensive care	High dependency
GCS ≤ 8 (focal injury on CT)	Skull fracture
GCS 6 (diffuse injury on CT)	Decreased level of consciousness
Multiple injuries	Post-traumatic seizure

Early intubation is advised for all patients with severe head injury as it has been shown to reduce secondary brain injury. Other indications for endotracheal intubation are given in Table 3.4.

Table 3.4: Indications for endotracheal intubation.

Absent gag reflex
GCS < 8
GCS 9–12, and patient being transferred to another centre
To protect the lower airway from blood, vomit or obstruction due to facial fractures
To allow positive pressure ventilation for ventilatory insufficiency
Uncontrolled seizures
To permit hyperventilation in order to reduce ICP

Control of ICP

ICP should be routinely monitored on those patients with an abnormal CT scan on admission or those with two or more poor prognostic indicators (systolic BP < 90 mmHg, age > 40 years, localising signs present):

- Nurse 25–45° head-up (enhances venous drainage).

- Avoid coughing on the endotracheal tube, particularly at times of tracheal suctioning, by use of adequate sedation, analgesia and if necessary muscle relaxants.

- Avoid rises in intrathoracic pressure by passing a nasogastric tube to prevent gastric dilatation and splinting of the diaphragm.

- Use of mannitol or furosemide (frusemide) to decrease ICP.

- Hyperventilate for acute raised ICP to lower $PaCO_2$ to 4–4.5 kPa and subsequently to reduce intracranial blood volume (however, this is accompanied by decreased cerebral blood flow leading to ischaemia and secondary brain injury).

Maintenance of cerebral perfusion pressure (CPP)

- Treat shock aggressively (avoid dextrose). Hypotension is unlikely to be due to brain injury unless it is in the terminal stages. Ensure an adequate circulating blood volume with IV fluids and/or blood guided by central venous pressure monitoring, urine output or pulmonary artery occlusion pressure recordings. The goal is a euvolaemic patient.

- Use of inotropic agents such as noradrenaline or dobutamine to increase mean arterial pressure.

Reduction in cerebral metabolic rate for O$_2$

- Use of hypothermia (rarely used).

- Administration of barbiturate infusions. However, they may cause hypotension and subsequently reduce CPP in doses required for cerebral protection.

- Avoidance of seizures.

The use of steroids has not been proven to be of benefit and remains controversial.

Frequent reassessment, early consultation with a neurosurgeon and prevention of secondary brain injury are the most important features of the management.

Monitoring

- Standard ITU monitoring with ICP monitoring for severe head injury:
  - ECG.
  - temperature.
  - urine output.
  - pulse oximetry.
  - invasive (intra-arterial) blood pressure.
- Jugular bulb venous oxygen saturation (SjvO$_2$) in some centres.
  - global measure of brain oxygenation.
  - SjvO$_2$ < 55 or >75% associated with poor prognosis.
  - detects cerebral desaturation.
- ICP monitoring (see Chapter 6):
  - can allow for withdrawal of CSF to quickly reduce ICP if required.
  - also allows determination of CPP.
  - should be used for all patients with GCS < 8.
- EEG monitoring can be used to monitor the progress of the head injury.
  - 16-channel EEG is a sensitive indicator of inadequate cerebral perfusion.
  - allows detection and monitoring of treatment of seizures.

Complications

- Seizures: anticonvulsants, e.g. phenytoin.

- Gastric ulceration: H_2 receptor antagonists, sucralfate and early enteral feeding for prevention.

- Infection:

    - from open (compound) fracture or basal skull fracture.

    - antibiotics to prevent infection.

    - suspected meningitis.

- Thrombo-embolism:

    - DVT/PE prevention measures.

    - discuss timing of the use of anticoagulants post-head injury in view of the possibility of bleeding.

- Diabetes insipidus/SIADH.

- Disseminated intravascular coagulation.

- Intracranial haematomas or abscesses: surgical decompression.

Prognosis

Often there is little that can be done about the primary brain injury. Rapid treatment allows reduction of the secondary insult. Early neurosurgical input in conjunction with minimising the secondary insult will improve the prognosis as much as possible.

Cross-reference

Chapter 2, p. 39. CSiG

Further reading

BF Matta, DK Menon, Initial management of acute head injury. *Surgery* 1998; 16: 13–15. SURGERY

DK Menon, BF Matta, Intensive care for acute head injury. *Surgery* 1998; 16: 204–8. SURGERY

BF Matta, DK Menon, Monitoring the brain after severe head injury. *Surgery* 1998; 16: 16–19. SURGERY

ATLS® Student Course Manual (Chicago: American College of Surgeons, 1997). American College of Surgeons Committee on Trauma

Recent advances in the management of traumatic brain injury: Andrews PJD, Souter MT. *Current Practice in Critical Illness* (London: Chapman & Hall, 1996), 61–87.

SPINAL INJURY

The incidence of spinal injuries is 15 per million of the population per year in the UK. The key consideration is that of cord damage.

Definition

The functional level in spinal cord injury is the most distal intact functional dermatome and the most distal motor level where the majority of muscles function at a 'fair' level.

Causes and demographics

The injuries to the spinal cord can be caused by either direct or indirect injuries.

Civilian injuries tend to be closed (indirect) injuries from violence to the vertebral column resulting in spinal cord injury. Military injuries are more commonly open (direct), most often from projectiles (bombs, shrapnel).

About 50% of spinal injuries in the UK are as a result of road traffic accidents. Of the injuries, 40% are either domestic or industrial, and the majority of the remainder occur when taking part in sporting activities.

Spinal cord injury tends to affect the working population with 75% of cases in people < 40 years of age with 80% of those affected being male.

Of those injured, 60% are affected at the thoracic spine, 30% are lumbar and 10% cervical. The thoracolumbar junction is particularly susceptible to injury as it forms a fulcrum to increased motion.

The type of force applied through the vertebral column affects the outcome:

- Compression: force applied in straight line, e.g. burst fractures: parachute injuries, falls from height.

- Distraction: e.g. chance fracture: seatbelt injury; hangman's fracture: neck hyperextension.

- Shearing: translation or rotation injuries: motorcycle and horse-riding accidents.

Classification and pathophysiology

Clinical classification of the fracture is important in patient management:

- Stable: spinal cord is rarely damaged, movement is safe.

- Unstable: cord is either damaged or may potentially be damaged by subsequent movement.

10% of fractures are unstable. Stability depends on both fracture pattern and associated ligamentous injury.

An alternative classification is based on cord injury:

- Cord concussion (neuropraxia):
    - flaccid motor paralysis, sensory loss, visceral paralysis below level of injury.
    - rapid complete recovery beginning within 8 h.
- Cord transection:
    - spinal shock initially (motor and visceral paralysis, sensory loss).
    - subsequent reflex activity below level of injury.
    - flaccid paralysis becomes spastic.
    - irreparable injury.
- Root transection:
    - motor and visceral paralysis and sensory loss in distribution of damaged nerve roots.
    - regeneration theoretically possible.
    - motor paralysis remains flaccid.
- Cord syndromes:
    - Central Cord Syndrome: hyperextension injury in the elderly with pre-existing cervical spondylosis:
        - upper limb paralysis.
        - central grey matter injured.
    - Anterior Cord Syndrome (poor prognosis):
        - paralysis, loss of pain sensation.
        - preservation of touch and joint position.
        - damage to anterior two-thirds of cord, sparing dorsal column.
    - Brown–Séquard syndrome:
        - ipsilateral paralysis.
        - contralateral loss of pain sensation.

Cord injuries are often regarded as complete or incomplete. Complete lesions have no function below the injured level. Incomplete lesions have some sparing of distal function.

Clinical

Resuscitate

- Airway + cervical spine control:
    - in-line immobilisation of cervical spine.
    - jaw thrust or chin lift.
    - collar, sand bags and taping (two-point).
- Breathing.
- Circulation.

Avoid further damage

- Spinal care:
    - hard collar and maintenance of alignment.
    - keep flat.
    - spinal lifting and log rolling.
- Spinal immobilisation:
    - cervical spine: collar halo vest/traction.
    - thoracolumbar spine: bracing/casting.

Surgery (specialist unit)

Indications are:

- Cord compression with progression of symptoms.
- Stabilisation of unstable fracture.

Prevention of complications

- Skin care (pressure sores): turn patient every 2 h, cleaning skin and meticulously smoothing sheets. Remove spinal board as soon as possible.
- Chest physiotherapy (respiratory tract infections) ± ventilatory support.
- Limb physiotherapy (prevent joint contractures).
- Bladder drainage (prevent reflux ± UTI), rectal disimpaction, bladder retraining.
- Antithrombotic therapy (DVT).

- Antacids/H$_2$ blockers (GI bleeds from stress ulceration).
- Nutrition.
- Counselling: restore self confidence; impotence.

Autonomic disturbance

- Decreased sympathetic tone causing peripheral vasodilation leads to:
  - decreased blood pressure.
  - decreased temperature.
  - decreased heart rate (lesions above T4 (cardiac accelerator fibres)).
- High-dose methylprednisolone (controversial) within 8 h.
- Anticoagulation 24 h after injury + TED stockings.

Respiratory

- High lesions → intercostal muscle paralysis → paradox chest movement.
- Rely on diaphragmatic breathing.
- Reduces the ability to cough and clear secretions.
- Increased risk of chest infection.

Monitoring

- Blood pressure: high lesion → orthostatic hypotension.
- Haemoglobin: GI bleeds.
- Respiration: respiratory rate, vital capacity, O$_2$ saturation.

Complications

- Further damage/neurological progression.
- Pressure sores.
- Respiratory tract infections.
- Urinary tract infections.
- Joint contractures.
- DVT.
- GI bleed.
- Psychological problems.

- Malnutrition.

- Malunion and non-union.

- Chronic pain.

Prognosis

Complete injuries show an improvement of one nerve root level in 80% of cases. Of these, 20% show an improvement of a further two levels.

Cross-reference

Chapter 2, p. 42. CSiG

MR McClelland, G Tharion. Acute spinal cord injury. *Surgery* 1999; 17: 25–30. SURGERY

Further reading

Apley AG, Solomon L. *System of Orthopaedics and Fractures* (London: Butterworths, 1993).

Miller MD. *Review of Orthopaedics,* 2nd Ed (Philadelphia: W. B. Saunders, 1996).

SYSTEMIC INFLAMMATORY RESPONSE SYNDROME (SIRS) AND MULTI-ORGAN DYSFUNCTION SYNDROME (MODS)

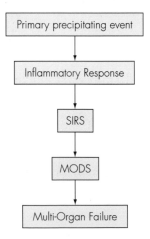

Figure 3.4: Pathway in the development of multi-organ failure.

Primary precipitating event

This follows tissue injury through infection, trauma, tumour invasion, hypoxia and ischaemia. The main causes are:

- Localised or generalised sepsis.

- Peritonitis (especially associated with pancreatitis).

- Burns.

- Trauma.

- Haemorrhage (particularly when associated with hypotension and hypoperfusion).

Secondary inflammatory process

The immune system is alerted to the threat posed by the tissue damage and reacts by instituting an inflammatory response to protect the body. This is exaggerated and subject to repeated positive feedback, leading to uncontrolled propagation by the inflammatory mediators involved. This results in endothelial cell damage and breakdown, causing the detrimental effects observed in SIRS.

This involves several inflammatory mediators (Table 3.5).

Table 3.5: Inflammatory mediators in SIRS.

Cytokines	Arachidonic acid derivatives	Stress hormones	Other mediators
Tumour necrosis factor (TNF)	Prostaglandins	Catecholamines	Histamine
Interleukins (IL-1, IL-6)	Leukotrienes	Steroids	Serotonin
Platelet activating factor (PAF)	Thromboxanes	Insulin	Bradykinin

The diagnosis of SIRS is made by the patient fulfilling two or more of the following criteria:

- Core temperature > 38 or < 36°C.

- Heart rate > 90 beats min^{-1}.

- Respiratory rate > 20 breaths min^{-1} or PaCO$_2$ < 4.26 kPa (32 mmHg).

- WCC > 12 × 10^9 litre^{-1} or < 4 × 10^9 litre^{-1} (with > 10% neutrophils or immature forms).

GIT bacterial translocation and the transfer of endotoxin via the hepatic portal venous system may be an important factor as a constant triggering mechanism in the propagation of this exaggerated response.

Nitric oxide (NO), also referred to as endothelium-derived relaxing factor (EDRF), is involved in the tonic relaxation of vascular smooth muscle, opposing the myogenic contraction of the vessel walls. With the onset of SIRS, the homeostasis of vascular tone is altered, and NO-mediated vasodilatation predominates, leading to the clinical effects seen in this condition.

Clinical effects of SIRS

These will vary depending on the precipitating cause and degree of involvement. There may be:

- Overt or occult infection.

- Flushed, warm peripheries.

- Hypotension (particularly diastolic).

- Tachycardia.

- Hypoxia.

- Metabolic acidosis on ABG (due to hypoperfusion and lactic acid accumulation).

- Deranged clotting function (since the coagulation cascade may be involved in the inflammatory response).

MODS

This is a progression from SIRS, resulting in end-organ dysfunction. It is diagnosed by dysfunction of two or more organ systems. The inflammatory process results in hypoperfusion and ischaemia of the tissues. The clinical picture will depend on the organ systems affected:

- Respiratory: often involved since they receive all of the cardiac output. Acute lung injury (ALI) and ARDS may occur following SIRS. The patient will be hypoxic and show signs and symptoms of respiratory failure (see Chapter 2).

- Cardiovascular: endothelial damage leads to extraversation of fluid from the vessels into the interstitium leading to oedema. Vasodilatation of arteries and veins results in hypotension, resulting in tissue hypoxia and lactic acidosis. There may be myocardial dysfunction resulting from the direct effects of inflammation and circulating mediators or endotoxin (in sepsis).

- Renal: there is oliguria (< 0.5 ml kg^{-1} h^{-1} urine production) because of reduced renal perfusion and filtration of inflammatory matter. Urea and creatinine may be elevated.

- Hepatic: hypoperfusion results in reduced metabolism of drugs and hormones, poor control of glucose homeostasis, synthetic failure, e.g. coagulation factors and failure to conjugate bilirubin (jaundice). The immunological role of the liver may be compromised reducing the ability to detoxify translocated bacteria from the GIT, thereby worsening SIRS. Tests of extrinsic coagulation and liver function may be abnormal.

- GIT: hypoperfusion and ischaemia results in atrophy. This increases the risk of bacterial translocation, thereby continuously triggering the inflammatory response.

- Cerebral: there may be confusion, sedation or agitation.

- Haematological. There may be anaemia, thrombocytopenia, leucopenia or leucocytosis. The tests of coagulation may show a range of abnormalities from prolonged intrinsic (APPT) and extrinsic (PT) clotting times to frank Disseminated Intravascular Coagulopathy (DIC).

If MODS is allowed to continue unchecked, then the organ dysfunction will become irreversible. At this stage, MOF is said to have occurred. This progression is potentially avoidable with appropriate treatment.

Management of MODS

The treatment aims are to support the organ systems affected, and to improve tissue perfusion and oxygenation.

Optimisation of oxygen delivery (DO_2) to the tissues

$$DO_2 = CO \times (1.34 \times Hb \times Sat/100) + \text{dissolved fraction,}$$

where $CO = SV \times HR$ and $BP = SVR \times CO$.

DO_2 can be maximised by maintaining adequate:

- Preload (fluid optimisation $\uparrow$ SV).

- Afterload (α-agonists $\uparrow$ SVR).

- Inotropic function (β-agonists $\uparrow$ SV).

- Chronotropic function (β-agonists $\uparrow$ HR).

- Haemoglobin concentration (> 10 g dl^{-1}).

- Haemoglobin saturation ($> 94\%$). This may require mechanical ventilation.

Searching for and treating sources of sepsis

These may be the primary precipitating cause or secondary colonisation in an immunocompromised host. Despite the active inflammatory response, the body's ability to deal with infection is low. The use of routine antibiotics cannot be recommended. Frequent tissue samples should be cultured and antimicrobial therapy directed at positively identified pathogens. In overwhelming or partially treated infection, positive cultures may be impossible to isolate. Blind therapy should be instituted only with the close involvement of the microbiology department. Inappropriate therapy may generate resistant strains and make current treatment more difficult.

Urine Output

Maintain an adequate urine output (> 0.5 ml kg^{-1} h^{-1}). Haemofiltration may be required (see Chapter 3, Renal replacement therapy).

Nutrition

Prevention of malnutrition. These patients have increased energy requirements since they are catabolic with greatly increased demand for substrate (see Chapter 3 Nutrition).

Prognosis

The risk of mortality depends on many factors:

- Age.
- Premorbid health.
- Severity of disease.
- Presence of sepsis.
- Number of organ systems affected and the duration of failure (Table 3.6).

Table 3.6: Mortality rates in MOF.

Number of failed organ systems	Mortality rate (%) on first day of organ failure	Mortality rate (%) on fourth day of organ failure
2	50	65
3	80	95

Cross-reference

Chapter 2, p. 37. CSiG

ACUTE RENAL FAILURE

The kidney is susceptible to the effects of underperfusion and hypoxaemia. This occurs most often in the context of MODS or SIRS (see above), but may be an isolated complication. The prevalence in ITU patients varies between 3 and 30%.

Definition

A rapid deterioration in renal function, especially Glomerular Filtration Rate (GFR), resulting in the accumulation of nitrogenous end products of metabolism, lasting days or weeks.

Classification

- Prerenal:

    - failure to perfuse the kidneys with blood. Renal function returns to normal once renal perfusion is restored.

    - Causes: dehydration, hypovolaemia, impaired cardiac function.

- Renal (intrinsic)

- Perfusion: secondary to prerenal causes (hypotension, hepatorenal syndrome, sepsis via decreased systemic vascular resistance):

    - glomerular: acute glomerulonephritis.

    - tubular: acute tubular necrosis (commonest), acute interstitial nephritis.

- Post-renal (obstruction)

- Within lumen: calculus, clot, tumour:

    - within wall: stricture.

    - outside wall: aneurysm, tumour, ureteric ligation, retroperitoneal fibrosis.

A patient may have renal failure due to more than one of the above categories.

Pathophysiology

Most cases are multifactorial.

- Renal cortical and medullary ischaemia.

- An alteration in glomerular haemodynamic factors:

    - decreased effective surface area for filtration.

    - reduced glomerular blood flow.

- decreased glomerular capillary permeability (secondary to endothelial cell swelling).

- Tubular abnormalities.

- Flow obstruction due to casts.

- Reverse leakage of glomerular ultrafiltrate.

Tubular effects are the more important in maintaining acute renal failure.

Diagnosis

- Progressive rise in serum urea and creatinine (only when > 50% glomerular function is lost).

- May be accompanied by:

  - oliguria (urine output < 0.5 ml kg^{-1} h^{-1}) (see Oliguria).

  - metabolic acidosis.

  - hyperkalaemia.

  - sodium and water retention (oedema).

Clinical

Investigations (Table 3.7).

Urinalysis and microscopy

- Urinalysis:

  - haematuria: glomerulonephritis.

  - proteinuria: glomerular/tubular disease.

  - glycosuria: tubular disease if blood glucose normal.

- Specific gravity:

  - concentrated: prerenal.

  - isotonic: parenchymal/obstructive.

- Casts:

  - hyaline: prerenal.

  - epithelial: acute tubular necrosis.

  - RBC: glomerulonephritis.

  - WBC (containing eosinophils): acute interstitial nephritis.

Urine biochemistry

- Creatinine clearance: reduced Na:Cr clearance ratio: prerenal. Assesses overall severity.

- Urine Na+, K+.

Bloods

- Urea and electrolytes: rising urea, creatinine, potassium.

- Electrophoresis: to exclude myeloma.

- FBC: eosinophilia: vasculitis.

  - Fragmentation of RBC: intravascular haemolysis.

- Arterial blood gases: metabolic acidosis.

Radiology

- Ultrasound scan: renal size, assess hydronephrosis/obstruction, assess bladder.

- AXR: assess renal size and parenchymal calcification.

- IVU: rarely indicated.

- CT: retroperitoneal fibrosis, ureteric obstruction.

Table 3.7: Laboratory investigations in acute renal failure.

	Normal	Prerenal	Renal	Post-renal
CVP		↓	↓,↑ or normal	↓,↑ or normal
Oliguria		✓	✓	✓
Haematuria		×	✓	✓
Serum urea	< 7.5	↑↑	↑↑	↑↑↑
Serum creatinine	3.5–125	↑	↑	↑
Serum U:Cr ratio		↑	normal	↑
Urine specific gravity	1.000–1.040	> 1.020	< 1.010	1.010
Urine osmolality (mosmol l⁻¹)	400–1400	> 500	285–295	260–330
Urine Na²⁺ (mmol l⁻¹)*		< 20	> 40	
Urine K⁺ (mmol l⁻¹)			< 10	
Proteinuria		×	✓	
Urine: plasma osmolality*	> 1.5	> 2	iso-osmolar	iso-osmolar
Urine: plasma urea*	> 20	> 30	< 10	< 5
Urine: plasma creatinine*		> 15	< 10	
Creatinine clearance	90–120	normal/↓	↓	↓
Fractional Na²⁺ excretion**		< 1	> 2	> 2

*May be affected by diuretic administration.
**FE Na = [urine Na × plasma Cr × 100]/[plasma Na × urine Cr].

Principles of treatment

A multidisciplinary approach involving both nephrologist and intensivist is desirable.

- Correct hyperkalaemia:

    - > 6 mmol l^{-1}: insulin 15 units + dextrose 50 ml/50%.

    - > 7 mmol l^{-1}: calcium gluconate 10–20 ml 10% + renal replacement therapy.

- Correct hypovolaemia ± hypotension and maintain intravascular volume.

- Prevent or correct volume overload (optimise fluid balance).

- Relieve urinary obstruction: urinary catheter, percutaneous nephrostomy, JJ stent.

- Treat underlying cause.

- Avoid further renal insults and nephrotoxic drugs (aminoglycosides, cisplatin, methotrexate, NSAIDs).

- Nutritional support (see Nutrition in the critically ill): ARF is a catabolic state so protein rich nutritional support is necessary.

- Treat uraemia by renal replacement therapy (see Renal replacement therapy).

Specifics of treatment

- Aim:

    - normovolaemia.

    - normotension (patient-specific).

    - diuresis (urine output maintained with inotropes and diuretics).

- Drugs:

    - dopamine 0.5–3 mcg kg^{-1} min^{-1}.

        - renal vasodilator →↑ RBF and GFR.

        - causes diuresis by ↓ Na$^+$ reabsorption →↑ Na$^+$ excretion.

    - Diuretics:

        - decrease intravascular volume.

        - decrease in renal O$_2$ consumption.

- Renal replacement therapy (see below):
  - indicated for uraemia, sodium/water overload, severe hyperkalaemia, urea > 30–50 mmol l⁻¹, creatinine > 0.7–1.5 mmol l⁻¹, HCO_3^- < 12 mmol l⁻¹.
  - haemodialysis.
  - peritoneal dialysis.
  - haemofiltration (CVVH) and haemodiafiltration (CVVH-D).

Monitoring

- Central venous pressure ± pulmonary artery occlusion pressure.
- Fluid balance (input/output).
- Electrolytes and electrolyte clearance.
  - Possible abnormalities:
    - ↑ potassium.
    - ↑ phosphate.
    - ↑ magnesium.
    - ↓ calcium.
- Arterial blood gases: metabolic acidosis.
- Urine osmolality.
- Electrocardiogram (hyperkalaemia: peaked T waves, small P, prolonged QRS Figure 1.7).

Complications

- Uraemic syndrome (uraemia = high serum urea): symptom complex associated with renal failure. Life-threatening manifestations are encephalopathy and pericarditis.
  - GI disturbances: stomatitis, nausea, vomiting.
  - CNS: confusion, disorientation, twitchy, convulsions.
  - acute uraemic fibrous pericarditis leading to cardiac tamponade.
  - haemopoietic disturbances and coagulopathies.
  - infection.
  - encephalopathy leading to respiratory failure.
- Chronic renal failure.
- Infection.
  - Risk factors: uraemia, dialysis catheter.

Prognosis

ARF has a high mortality of 30–80%. This is increased in ITU patients to 60–80%. Burns patients with ARF have a mortality rate of 75%. Prognosis is poorest when ARF is part of MODS and also after GI surgery.

See also Chapter 3, Oliguria, and Renal replacement therapy.

Cross-reference

Madden BP. Clinical assessment of renal function. *Surgery* 2000; SURGERY 18: 135–8.

Raftery AT. Renal failure: diagnosis, management and dialysis. SURGERY *Surgery* 1999; 17: 208–12.

Further reading

Gesualdo L *et al.* Acute renal failure in critically ill patients. *Intensive Care Medicine* 1999; 25: 1188–90.

OLIGURIA

Definition

- Urine output < 0.5 ml kg^{-1} h^{-1}.

Causes

- Blocked catheter: check with bladder washout.
- All causes of acute renal failure (see Acute Renal Failure).
- All causes of shock (see Chapter 1, Management of haemorrhage and shock).

Classification and pathophysiology

Oliguria is usually the first manifestation of renal impairment.

Clinical

Investigations

- Renal function studies (Table 3.7):
  - urinalysis: ↑ specific gravity.
  - osmolarity: urine and plasma: these measurements are affected by early furosemide (frusemide) administration.
  - osmolality: low is indicative of failure of kidney to concentrate urine.
  - fractional sodium excretion (F_{Na} < 1%: volume depletion).
  - urea.
  - 24-h creatinine clearance.
- Radiology: ultrasound scan – to exclude obstructive causes.

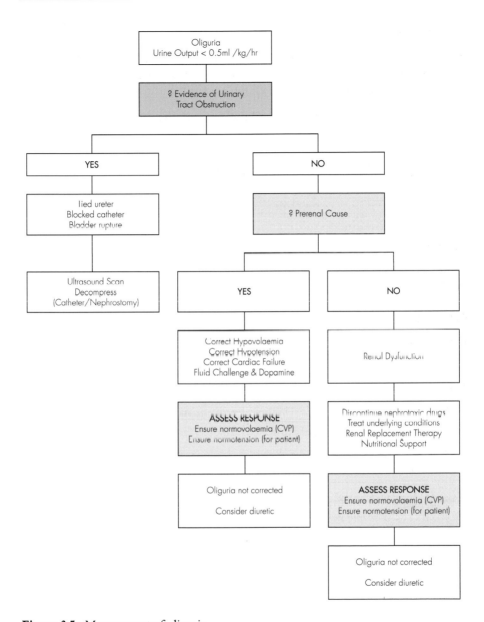

Figure 3.5: Management of oliguria.

If oliguria persists, crystalloid intake should be reduced and drug doses reviewed.

Monitoring

- Accurate fluid balance chart (hourly).
- Urea and electrolytes (hyperkalaemia).
- Arterial blood gases: acidosis.

Complications

Rapid and effective resuscitation and the avoidance of nephrotoxic drugs (NSAIDs especially) reduce the incidence of complications. Early introduction of haemofiltration may be necessary (see Renal replacement therapy):

- Acute renal failure.
- Hyperkalaemia.

RENAL REPLACEMENT THERAPY

Haemodialysis

Definition

The process of separating crystalloids and colloids in solution by the difference in rates of diffusion through a semipermeable membrane.

Pathophysiology

Haemodialysis rapidly clears urea and creatinine. It involves the movement of large fluid volumes between compartments. Therefore, it carries risk in haemodynamically unstable patients. Its principal usage is in chronic renal failure.

There are four major controlling factors in haemodialysis:

- Blood flow rate.
- Membrane permeability.
- Dialysis duration.
- Transmembrane pressure.

Indications

Table 3.8: Indications for haemodialysis.

Absolute	Relative
Increasing hyperkalaemia	Acute Renal Failure
Hypoxia secondary to fluid overload	
Acidosis	
Uraemia causing coma and/or pericarditis	

Complications

- Hypotension.

- GI bleed (H2 antagonist prophylaxis).

- Infection.

- Encephalopathy.

- Dialysis disequilibrium syndrome. This is the manifestation of central nervous systems symptoms and signs during or after dialysis.

Peritoneal dialysis

Definition

Dialysis occurring across the peritoneal membrane (dialysis through the abdominal wall within the peritoneal cavity).

Classification

There are three types of peritoneal dialysis:

- Acute Peritoneal Dialysis: fluid exchanges every 10–30 min. Used in the critical care setting.

- Continuous Ambulatory Peritoneal Dialysis (CAPD).

- Continuous Cyclical Peritoneal Dialysis (CCPD).

Both CAPD and CCPD involve longer cycle times and less frequent fluid exchanges. Usage of either is uncommon in the ITU setting.

Principles

The principle of peritoneal dialysis involves the instillation of dialysate fluid into the peritoneal cavity. This fluid remains *in situ* for a period of time to allow for diffusion of metabolites across the peritoneal membrane. The fluid is then drained and the cycle repeated.

Four key factors influence peritoneal dialysis quality:

- Thickness of or inflammation of the peritoneal membrane.
- Blood flow to the peritoneal lining.
- Size of the peritoneal cavity.
- Presence of infection.

Indications

The indications for patients unsuitable for haemodialysis are given in Table 3.9.

Table 3.9: Indications for peritoneal dialysis.

Absolute	Relative
Cerebral haemorrhage	Poor vascular access
Patient unsafe for anticoagulant therapy	Absence of a catabolic state
Severe congestive heart failure	

The usage of peritoneal dialysis (PD) in the critical care setting has reduced because of the advent of haemofiltration (see Haemofiltration and haemodiafiltration).

Contraindications

- Undiagnosed or untreated intra-abdominal disease.
- Recent or multiple abdominal surgical procedures (adhesions).
- Hypercatabolic states.
- Past medical history of peritonitis.

Access

PD requires access to the peritoneal cavity. This can be either:

- Rigid (single use) temporary catheter inserted either with or preferably without a trocar; or
- Silicon catheter with a Dacron cuff (Tenckhoff), which is inserted for long-term use.

Monitoring

General biochemical monitoring is essential, with close observation of:

- Potassium (hypokalaemia).
- Glucose (absorbed from the dialysate).
- Albumin (marked protein loss is possible).

Complications

- Peritonitis: infective, usually *Staphylococcus epidermidis* or *S. aureus*.

- Ileus.

- Indigestion/shortness of breath.

- Complications of increased intra-abdominal pressure: herniae, dialysate leakage from catheter site.

- Acute hydrothorax: undetected diaphragmatic defect.

- Protein deficiency: protein loss into dialysate.

Haemofiltration and haemodiafiltration

Principles

Haemofiltration (continuous venovenous haemofiltration, CVVH) has replaced continuous arteriovenous haemofiltration (CAVH), which produced varying ultrafiltrates dependent on the patient's arterial pressure.

The principle of CVVH is to:

- Remove the patient's blood.

- Pump it through the filter at a steady rate and pressure.

- Return the remaining venous blood to the circulation.

CVVH requires large volumes (> 500 ml h^{-1}) of ultrafiltrate to be produced to be effective in removing solute.

Haemodiafiltration (CVVH-D) relies on a countercurrent system (Figure 3.6). The benefits of this are:

- Improved solute clearance.

- Slower rate of ultrafiltration.

- Easier fluid balance management.

These benefits make CVVH-D the renal support therapy of choice in the critically ill.

Indications

The acutely ill, haemodynamically unstable patient in acute renal failure.

Intermittent haemofiltration can be used to remove large quantities of fluid in controlled circumstances, e.g. cardiopulmonary bypass (see Chapter 1, General principles of cardiopulmonary bypass).

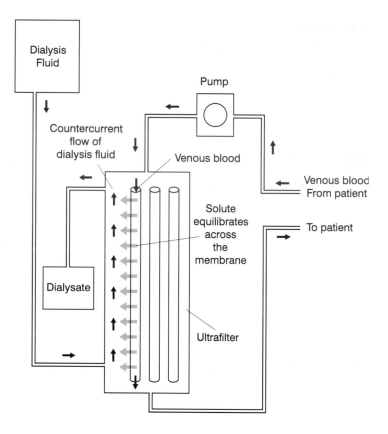

Figure 3.6: Principles of CVVH-D. (Reproduced from Fundamentals of Surgical Practice, GMM, 1998).

Complications

- Bleeding.
- Hypotension.
- Hypothermia.

Cross-reference

Chapter 38, p. 366.   CSiG

Further reading

Critical Care Secrets. Parsons PE, Wiener-Kronish JP, Hanley & Belfus (Philadelphia), 1992.

Fundamentals of Surgical Practice. Eds Aljafri Majid & Andrew Kingsnorth, Greenwich Medical Media (London) 1998.

GASTROINTESTINAL TRACT

Gastrointestinal haemorrhage

Acute GI bleeds are an important cause of mortality and morbidity. GI bleeds may occur as the primary pathology or as part of Multi-Organ Dysfunction Syndrome (see Multisystem failure and systemic inflammatory response syndrome). Protocols for managing severe GI bleeds are commonplace and enable identification of those patients with life-threatening bleeding and those at risk of rebleed.

Classification

- Primary: massive upper/lower GI haemorrhage.

- Secondary: multisystem, critically ill patients who develop secondary GI haemorrhage as a complication of their principal pathology.

Causes

Table 3.10: Causes of GI haemorrhage.

Upper GI haemorrhage	Lower GI haemorrhage
Peptic ulcer disease	Colorectal carcinoma
Gastritis	Polyps
Stress ulceration	Ischaemic colitis
Oesophagitis	Inflammatory bowel disease
Oesophageal varices	Diverticular disease
	Angiodysplasia

Clinical

The rate and pattern of bleeding depends on the underlying cause. Clinical features to be looked for include:

- Shock.

- Haematemesis, melaena.

- Fresh blood per rectum.

- Pain.

- Vomiting.

Baseline investigations include:

- Haematology: FBC, clotting, Hct, crossmatch.

- Biochemistry: U&E, LFT.

- Radiology: AXR, CXR.

- Special investigations:

  - OGD (upper GI endoscopy), sigmoidoscopy, colonoscopy.

  - angiography (very accurate: detects bleeding 0.5–1 ml min^{-1}).

- A nasogastric tube should be inserted to ascertain the presence of blood in the stomach.

Treatment

- Resuscitate (ABC):

  - restore volume.

  - oxygenate.

- Secondary treatment depends on underlying cause (Table 3.11).

Table 3.11: Treatment of selected causes of GI bleeds.

Diagnosis	Treatment options
Oesophageal varices	Sengstaken–Blakemore tube, sclerotherapy, vasopressin, TIPS (transjugular intrahepatic portosystemic shunt), surgery
Peptic ulcer disease	H2 antagonist/proton pump inhibitor, OGD + inject, surgery
Lower GI bleeds	selective angiography and ablation, OGD+ injection/cautery/polypectomy/laser coagulation, surgery

Indications for surgery

- Surgically amenable cause identified.

- Unstable patient despite aggressive resuscitation (6–8 unit transfusion).

- Second rebleed within 48 h.

Complications

- Rebleed: especially bad in the elderly and those with chronic diseases (hypertension, cardiac and renal failure, cirrhosis).

- Hepatic failure (see Chapter 3, hepatic failure): blood in GI tract results in raised urea and ammonia and causes deterioration in mental function.

Prognosis

- Early aggressive resuscitation reduces mortality rate.

- Upper GI bleeds requiring > 10 units transfusion are associated with ~30% mortality rate.

Cross reference

Parvanta L, Allum WH. Gastrointestinal haemorrhage.
Surgery 1999; 17: 293–8.

SURGERY

Spencer J. Colonic haemorrhage. *Surgery* 1998; 16: 61–5.

SURGERY

Acute pancreatitis

Acute pancreatitis has an annual incidence of ~50–200 per million of the UK population.

Definition

An acute, potentially reversible inflammation of the pancreas, with significant mortality and morbidity.

Classification

- Severity: Glasgow criteria (Table 3.12). One point scored for each criterion present. A score of ≥ 2 indicates a severe attack.

Table 3.12: Modified Glasgow (Imrie) criteria for severity of acute pancreatitis.

Criterion	Within 48 h of admission
Age	> 55
WCC	> 15 × 10^9
Plasma/serum urea	> 16 mmol l^{-1}
Glucose	> 10 mmol l^{-1} (unless diabetic)
Plasma/serum Ca^{2+}	< 2 mmol l^{-1}
Plasma/serum albumin	< 32 g l^{-1}
PaO$_2$	< 8 kPa
Plasma/serum LDH	> 600 iu l^{-1}

- Aetiological: see causes.
- Morphological:
  - oedematous: mild.
  - necrotising: severe.

Diagnosis

- Serum amylase > 1000 iu l^{-1} (or 3× upper limit of laboratory normal).
- Urinary amylase remains elevated longer than serum amylase.
- Serum lipase more sensitive, specific and difficult to do/obtain.

Causes

Gallstones and alcohol account for 70% of acute pancreatitis in the UK.

- Obstructive:
  - gallstones.
  - afferent loop obstruction post-gastric surgery.
- Toxins:
  - alcohol.
  - scorpion venom (ampullary spasm).
- Metabolic:
  - hypercalcaemia and hyperparathyroidism.
  - hyperlipidaemia.
  - diabetic ketoacidosis.
- Drugs:
  - thiazide diuretics.
  - furosemide (frusemide).
  - tetracyclines and many more.
- Iatrogenic:
  - post-ERCP.
  - post-abdominal surgery.
- Miscellaneous:
  - infection: mumps, Epstein–Barr virus.
  - trauma: handlebar injury.

Pathophysiology

The principal pathophysiological feature is of autodigestion (proteolysis) by activated enzymes, leading to necrosis.

It is thought duodenopancreatic reflux is a mechanism for this.

The remote organ system dysfunction is mediated by inflammatory responses to leucocyte derived cytokines.

Clinical

- Signs and symptoms: severe abdominal pain radiating to the back, nausea and vomiting, epigastric tenderness. Grey Turner's sign (grey discoloration of the flanks) and Cullen's sign (periumbilical discoloration).

- Management: UK guidelines are to promote early diagnosis and clinical vigilance to detect complications.

- Investigations:

  - amylase ($\pm$ lipase).

  - contrast enhanced CT or MRI: suggests causes (gallstones, liver metastases), assesses severity (pancreatic enlargement and localised fluid collections).

  - ultrasound abdomen/biliary tree (identifies gallstones).

Treatment

- Nasogastric tube/nil by mouth: drains stomach and rests gut.

- Fluid replacement: CVP or pulmonary artery catheter may be necessary to gauge fluid replacement.

- Control symptoms: analgesia (consider epidural), anti-emetic.

- Metabolic support: correct $\downarrow Ca^{2+}$, $\downarrow Mg^{2+}$, $\uparrow$ glucose.

- Nutritional support: TPN (see Nutrition in the critically ill).

- Surgery for debridement of infected pancreatic necrosis with subsequent drainage of pancreatic bed.

- Prevention of complications: prophylaxis against GI haemorrhage.

- Antibiotics: if infection present.

Monitoring

- Respiratory rate.

- Urine output.

- Arterial blood gases: hypoxia.

- Biochemistry: hypocalcaemia.

- Glucose.

- White count: neutrophilia.

Complications

Management of life-threatening complications has been addressed by new UK guidelines (Table 3.13).

Table 3.13: UK guidelines for the management of life-threatening complications of acute pancreatitis (Atlanta and Santorini Symposia). From British Society of Gastroenterology, United Kingdom guidelines for the management of acute pancreatitis *Gut* 1998; 42 (suppl. 2): S1–13.

	Incidence rate (%)	Mortality rate (%)	Criterion	Mechanism/ treatment
Organ system failure				
Respiratory failure	20	25	$PaO_2 < 8$ kPa	pulmonary oedema with impaired gas exchange → ARDS. Rx: early PEEP
Renal failure	5	65	serum creatinine > 177 μmol l^{-1}	hypovolaemia + splanchnic vasoconstriction
Cardiovascular failure	5	90	systolic BP < 90 mmHg	endothelia damage → capillary leakage → hypovolaemia: high output shock
Metabolic disturbance			$Ca^{2+} < 1.87$ mmol l^{-1}	
GI haemorrhage			haemorrhage > 500 ml 24 h^{-1}	prophylaxis
Pancreatic collections				
Necrosis				debridement of solid infected necrosis
Abscess				surgical/percutaneous drainage
Acute pseudocyst				cystogastrostomy

- Multiple organ failure (see Multisystem Failure and systemic inflammatory response syndrome).

- Single system organ failure (Table 3.13).

- DIC (see Chapter 1, Disseminated intravascular coagulopathy).

- Chronic pancreatitis.

- Deep venous thrombosis.

- Hyperglycaemia.

Prognosis

Major local or systemic complications occur in 20% of cases with death in 10%, the commonest cause of death being pancreatic infection.

Increasing severity of complications and multiple organ failure carry the highest mortality rate (Table 3.14).

Table 3.14: Incidence and mortality rates of multiple organ failure.

	Incidence rate (%)	Mortality rate (%)
Single system organ failure	20	20
Double system organ failure	4	55
Triple system organ failure	1.5	90

Cross-reference

Larvin M, Acute pancreatitis. *Surgery* 1999; 17: 261–5.   SURGERY

Hepatic failure
Definition

Acute liver failure arising as a consequence of extensive necrosis of liver cells resulting in impairment of liver function and hepatic encephalopathy.

Classification

Two major classifications are used (Table 3.15).

Table 3.15: Classifications of hepatic failure.

Classification		
Onset of encephalopathy after jaundice	hyperacute	0–7 days
	acute	8–28 days
	subacute	29 days–12 weeks
Alternative	fulminant	massive necrosis of liver cells or other sudden severe impairment of hepatic function
	late onset	encephalopathy 8–26 weeks after onset of symptoms
	acute on chronic	acute illness causes decompensation of pre-existing chronic liver disease (usually cirrhosis)
	ischaemia	secondary to cardiac failure or shock

Diagnosis

- Coagulation defect: INR > 2.0.

- ↑ Hepatic enzymes (AST and ALT).

- Prothrombin concentration < 50% of normal in the presence of features of acute liver failure.

Causes

- Viral infection:

  - hepatitis A–G.

  - varicella zoster and herpes simplex more rarely.

- Drugs:

  - paracetamol.

  - halothane.

  - ethanol.

- Ischaemia.

- MODS (see Multisystem failure and systemic inflammatory response syndrome).

- Miscellaneous causes in an already diseased liver:

  - GI bleed.

  - infection.

- electrolyte imbalance: diuretics/rapid drainage ascites.

- surgery and trauma.

- ethanol and narcotics.

Pathophysiology

The major pathological process is massive coagulative necrosis of liver cells.

Clinical

- Jaundice.

- Hepatic encephalopathy: four stages:

  I. altered mood: prodrome.

  II. increasing drowsiness.

  III. stupor.

  IV. deep coma.

- Cerebral oedema.

- Coagulopathy:

  - decreased synthesis of clotting factors V, VII, IX, X.

  - thrombocytopenia

  - GI bleed.

- Metabolic derangement:

  - hypoglycaemia.

  - metabolic alkalosis.

  - lactic acidosis.

- Electrolyte imbalance:

  - hypokalaemia: inadequate intake, vomiting.

  - hyponatraemia: H_2O retention.

  - hypomagnesaemia.

  - hypocalcaemia.

  - hypophosphataemia.

- Respiratory failure and ARDS.

- Sepsis.

Investigations

- Serology.

- Drug screen.

- As per monitoring (Table 3.17).

Treatment

Early transfer to a specialist unit is recommended.

The main principles of the treatment of acute liver failure are supportive care and the identification of potential transplant recipients:

- Reverse precipitating factors: GI bleed, renal failure.

- Oral lactulose.

- Decrease dietary protein.

- Control infection: consider selective decontamination of the gut (neomycin).

- Support other systems:

    - fluid replacement: 5% dextrose is the fluid of choice.

    - inotropes for CVS.

    - mechanical ventilation ± PEEP for RS.

- Mannitol 0.5g kg^{-1} ± furosemide (frusemide) for cerebral oedema.

- Transplant (Table 3.16).

- Liver assist devices are undergoing studies at present.

Table 3.16: KCH criteria for offering transplants in liver failure.

Criteria for offering transplants in non-paracetamol induced liver failure (≥3 criteria need to be satisfied)
Age < 10 or > 40 years
Prothrombin time > 50 s
Non-A–non-B hepatitis/drug induced hepatitis
Bilirubin > 300 μmol l^{-1}
Jaundice to encephalopathy time > 7 days
or
Prothrombin time > 100 s

Modified from Surgery 1999 (The Medicine Publishing Group, Oxon) with permission.

Monitoring

See Table 3.17.

Table 3.17: Monitoring in acute hepatic failure.

Continuous	6 Hourly	12 Hourly	Daily
CVP	platelets	U&E	AST, Bil, ALP, ALT
Arterial pressure	clotting (PT/INR)	Hb, WBC	albumin
O₂ saturation	glucose	ABG	CXR
Urine output			ECG
Temperature			
ICP monitor*			

*ICP monitoring in patients with coagulopathy has a 5% risk of intracranial bleed.

Complications

- Upper GI haemorrhage: oesophagitis, gastric erosions, duodenal ulcer.

- Infection:

    - Gram +ve and −ve anaerobes.

    - respiratory tract infections.

    - urinary tract infections.

    - fungal infections after 1 week.

    - sepsis increases liver dysfunction and often leads to death.

Prognosis

Acute hepatic failure has a high mortality rate with an overall survival rate of ~20%, increased to 70% by transplant.

Prognosis is influenced by age, grade of encephalopathy, bilirubin level and creatinine concentration. Metabolic acidosis confers an extremely poor prognosis.

Death is usually due to cerebral oedema and sepsis.

Cross-reference

Heaton ND, Prachalias AA. Principles and current status of liver transplantation. *Surgery* 1999; 17: 216–19. SURGERY

NUTRITION IN THE CRITICALLY ILL

It is essential to provide the critically ill patient with the necessary nutrients to repair damaged tissues and preserve defence mechanisms.

Table 3.18: Fluid and electrolyte composition of the body.

	Intracellular fluid (ICF)	Extracellular water (ECF)		Daily requirement
		Interstitial fluid	Plasma volume	
Volume of water (litres)	25	14	3*	35 ml kg^{-1}
Na$^+$ (mmol l^{-1})	10	143	140	1–2 mmol kg^{-1}
K$^+$ (mmol l^{-1})	155	3.8	3.7	1–2 mmol kg^{-1}
Ca^{2+} (mmol l^{-1})	< 0.01	1.2	1.2	0.17 mmol kg^{-1}
Mg^{2+} (mmol l^{-1})	2	0.8	0.7	0.15 mmol kg^{-1}
PO$_4^{3-}$ (mmol l^{-1})	100	1.1	1.1	0.5 mmol kg^{-1}
Cl$^-$ (mmol l^{-1})	3	114	101	
HCO$_3^-$ (mmol l^{-1})	10	30	27	

*Total blood volume = plasma volume (3 litres) + cell volume (2 litres) = 5 litres.

Table 3.19: Composition of commonly used crystalloid infusions.

(mmoll^{-1})	Physiological saline (0.9%)	Hartmann's solution	Dextrose (4%) Saline (0.18%)	5% Dextrose
Na$^+$	155	131	30	0
K$^+$	0	5	0	0
Ca^{2+}	0	2	0	0
Cl$^-$	155	111	30	0
HCO$_3^-$	0	29*	0	0
Osmolality (mosmol kg^{-1})	308	308		278
Distribution in body water	ECF	ECF	0.5 ICF, 0.5 ECF	TBW

*This is in the form of lactate, which is metabolised in the liver to bicarbonate.
The osmolality of blood is 290 mosmol kg^{-1}.

Fluid replacement

This depends on from which body compartment the fluid is lost. Replace like with like (Table 3.20).

Table 3.20: Replacement of fluid losses.

Fluid loss	Fluid replacement
Haemorrhage	Blood
Plasma, e.g. burns and peritonitis (especially in pancreatitis)	FFP or plasma substitute, e.g. colloids
Na^+ and H_2O (ECF), e.g. vomiting, diarrhoea and sweating	Normal saline
H_2O alone (TBW), e.g. diabetes insipidus	5% dextrose

General nutritional requirements

These depend on:

- Size → assessed by body mass index (BMI) (also known as the Quatelet index):

  BMI = weight (kg)/height^2 (m^2).

  Normally 20–25 (< 19 = malnourished).

- Premorbid nutritional status.

- Current clinical condition and metabolic demands.

Daily requirements

These are divided into protein and non-protein (carbohydrate and fat) energy. The proportions of these will vary depending on the individual needs of the patient. It should be noted that patients receiving infusions of propofol require less fat added to their feed:

  Nitrogen balance = intake – loss (g N day^{-1}).
  Intake = protein/6.25 (g N day^{-1}).

- Nitrogen requirement is 0.2g kg^{-1} day^{-1}.

- This is usually 9 g N day^{-1} for males; 7.5g N day^{-1} for females.

- In non-catabolic patients, this represents 1 g N per 200 kcal energy.

- In catabolic patients, this represents 1 g N per 80–100 kcal energy.

Glutamine is an essential amino acid and is important for wound healing and gluconeogenesis. It must be added to feed since it is unstable in solution.

Energy requirements are calculated from BMR: these are usually 20–30 kCal kg^{-1} day^{-1}:

- 2500 kCal for males.

- 2000 kCal for females.

Table 3.21: Variability in energy requirements.

↑ **Energy requirements**	↓ **Energy requirements**
Patients being conscious, sitting or ambulatory	patients being unconscious and sedated
Pyrexia	mechanical ventilation
Malnutrition	
Sepsis and burns	

Nutrition in organ failure

- Cardiac: ↓ Na^+ and ↓ H_2O (to ↓ fluid overload).

- Respiratory: ↑ fat and ↓ carbohydrate (to ↓ CO_2 production).

- Renal:

    - ↓ nitrogen (to ↓ urea production).

    - ↓ fat (poor handling).

    - ↓ H_2O and ↓ Na^+ (to ↓ fluid overload).

    - ↓ K^+ (to avoid hyperkalaemia).

- Liver:

    - ↓ H_2O and ↓ Na^+ (to ↓ fluid overload, particularly in ascites).

    - ↓ nitrogen (in encephalopathic patients).

    - adequate carbohydrate load (tend towards hypoglycaemia).

- Cerebral: close blood glucose control needed (main substrate), since hyperglycaemia worsens cerebral oedema.

- Stressed patient: limit glucose to 5g kg^{-1} day^{-1}.

Enteral nutrition

This can take many forms:

- Oral supplements.

- Enteral tube feeding:

    - nasogastric.

    - nasojejunal.

    - PEG (unusual in the critically ill).

    - PEJ (usually after surgery).

Advantages

- Cheap and simple to implement.
- No central venous access required.
  - ↓ risk of infection.
  - ↓ risk of mechanical complications of insertion.
- Maintains the physiological role of the GIT.
- ↑ GIT blood flow:
  - prevents breakdown of mucosal lining.
  - prevents translocation of GIT bacteria.
  - this may prevent the development of SIRS and MODS.
- Protects against stress ulceration.
- Early commencement (within the first 24 h):
  - ↓ ICU stay.
  - ↓ septic complications: this is especially true in multitrauma.

Disadvantages

- Need functioning GIT.
- ↑ Risk of nosocomial pneumonia.
- Delivery system (tubes) are source of morbidity:
  - nasal ulceration.
  - sinusitis.
  - traumatic removal (poorly tolerated by some patients).
  - tube occlusion.
  - displaced tubes.
  - peritonitis with percutaneous tubes.
  - bacterial colonisation.
- LOS dysfunction can lead to regurgitation and aspiration of feed.
- ↑ Incidence of diarrhoea.
- ↑ Incidence of nausea and vomiting.
- Malabsorption leads to malnourishment, which can be difficult to detect.
- Hyperglycaemia.

Signs of adequate GIT function

- Bowel sounds are notoriously unreliable as an indicator of GIT activity in the critically ill. Feed should not be commenced with tinkling BS or other signs of bowel obstruction.

- NG aspirate should ideally be < 50 ml h^{-1} (averaged over 4–6 h).

- Abdominal distension or pain should be referred for surgical opinion and evaluation, and the cause determined. There is a risk of abdominal distension with gas during assisted ventilation, particularly when the patient is being weaned and taking spontaneous breaths.

- Absence of defecation or the presence of diarrhoea are not good indicators for the success of enteral nutrition, but pre-existing diarrhoea is likely to be made worse with feeding.

Patients unsuitable for enteral nutrition

- Bowel obstruction.
- Anastomotic breakdown.
- GIT inflammation.
- GIT bleeding.
- GIT infection.

Regimen for enteral feeding

- Start at 10 ml h^{-1}.

- Increase to 30, 60, 90 and 120 ml h^{-1} every 12 h provided that gastric aspirate < 20 ml h^{-1} (averaged over several hours). If gastric aspirate is high then the infusion rate should be decreased or other measures used to prevent regurgitation of enteral feed:

  - use of nasoduodenal and nasojejunal feeding tubes.

  - use of prokinetic agents, e.g. metoclopromide, cisapride or erythromycin.

- There should be a rest period of between 4 and 6 h every day. This allows the gastric acidity to return towards normal, decreasing the risk of nosocomial pneumonia.

Parenteral nutrition

Advantages

- All of prescribed feed reaches the bloodstream.
- Rests damaged areas of the GIT.

Disadvantages

- Central venous access required:
  - invasive (for complications see Chapter 6 Vascular Access).
  - expertise needed.
  - infection risk.
- Expensive.
- Unphysiological:
  - fatty liver.
  - ↑ insulin requirements.
- GIT atrophy.

Routes of administration

- Peripheral: suitable for feeds with < 2000 kcal day^{-1} with < 14 g N. The main problem is with thrombophlebitis, the incidence of which may be reduced by:
  - ↓ osmolality of the feed.
  - ↑ fat content.
- Central:
  - long lines are usually sited via the basilic vein into the SCV. The main disadvantages are that the tip can be displaced during arm movement, and that a long line is uncomfortable for the conscious patient (who cannot bend the arm).
  - multilumen infusion catheters. Should be used for short periods (only up to 7 days) as they pose a high risk for infective complications. This is minimised by using a dedicated port for parenteral feed and careful asepsis when connecting new TPN bags.
  - tunnelled lines are the gold standard for prolonged parenteral feeding. They should be inserted with strict asepsis into a central vein, and are tunnelled subcutaneously to exit onto the anterior chest wall. They may be used for weeks to months.

Monitoring

- Daily biochemistry.
- Fluid balance.

- Nutritional status.

- Tube placement (X-ray).

Cross-reference

Chapter 11, p. 129. CSiG

Pennington CR. Nutritional support in surgery. *Surgery* 2000; SURGERY
18: 69–71.

MULTIPLE AND LIFE-THREATENING TRAUMA

Major trauma is responsible for > 10 000 deaths and 100 000 injuries per year in the UK. It is the leading cause of death in those < 40 years of age and is increasing in prevalence. The multidisciplinary ATLS® approach is employed in managing major trauma patients.

Causes

- Penetrating: knives, glass, fragments from explosives.

- Blast: bombs.

- Blunt: RTA.

- Deceleration: RTA, air crashes, falls, parachuting.

- Crush: mining, industrial, RTA, natural disasters.

- Miscellaneous: heat, cold, radiation, chemical, barotrauma.

Classification

- By cause (mechanism of injury) (see above).

- By body system involvement:

  - head and neck.

  - thoracic.

  - abdominal/pelvic.

  - limb/extremity.

  - multiple.

- By trauma severity scoring (see Chapter 5, Scoring and outcome measures):

- Abbreviated Injury Score (AIS).

- Injury Severity Score (ISS).

- Revised Trauma Score (RTS).

- TRISS (compound of RTS and ISS).

Pathophysiology

There is a trimodal death distribution following major trauma (Table 3.22).

Table 3.22: Trimodal death distribution in trauma.

Immediate (at scene)	Early (2–3 h)	Late (≥1 week)
Brain laceration	Hypoxia	Pulmonary embolus
Brainstem/high spinal cord injury	Haemorrhage	Sepsis
Heart/great vessel injury	Golden Hour aims to reduce these deaths	Multi-organ Dysfunction Syndrome (MODS)

The pathophysiological responses of the body are designed to maximise the chances of survival.

Early responses

- Neuroendocrine:

  - pituitary:

    - ↑ CRF secretion →↑ ACTH secretion →↑ cortisol.

    - ↑ growth hormone.

    - ↑ endorphins.

    - ↑ prolactin.

    - ↑ vasopressin.

    - ↑ sympathetic activity →↑ noradrenaline (norepinephrine) and adrenaline (epinephrine) from adrenal medulla.

- Metabolic:

  - stimulation of glycogenolysis and lipolysis → hyperglycaemia.

  - decreased glucose utilisation → potentiates hyperglycaemia.

- Protein:

    - ↑ CRP.

    - ↑ fibrinogen.

- Thermoregulation: tissue injury → nociceptive impulses →↓ temperature.

- Cardiovascular: response to shock (see Chapter 1, Management of haemorrhage and shock):

    - ↑ heart rate.

    - ↑ peripheral vascular resistance.

Late responses

- Metabolic rate (Table 3.23).

Table 3.23: Alterations in metabolic rate in trauma.

Metabolic rate ↑ by	Post-trauma scenarios leading to ↓ metabolic rate
Injury	↓ food intake ↓ muscle mass ↓ O_2 supply

- there is an upward resetting of thermoregulation leading to increased sympathetic activity.

- catecholamine release leads to increased energy production.

- Protein and amino acid metabolism:

    - ↑ urinary N_2 output.

    - ↑ whole body protein turnover.

        - injury →↑ breakdown and ↑ synthesis.

        - undernutrition →↓ synthesis.

        - net effect ↑ protein breakdown (principally skeletal muscle).

- Carbohydrate metabolism:

    - hyperglycaemia.

    - inappropriately high plasma insulin.

    - overall picture: insulin resistance.

- Fat metabolism: ↓ non-esterified fatty acids.

Clinical

The key principles are:

- Access to care.

- Prehospital care and transfer to level 1 trauma centre.

- Resuscitation:

    - ATLS® principles:

        – Airway and cervical spine control.

        – Breathing and ventilation.

        – Circulation and haemorrhage control.

        – Disability.

        – Exposure.

    - Oxygenation (supra-normal O_2 delivery).

    - Ventilation.

    - Vascular access.

    - Shock management.

- Reassessment.

- Detailed secondary survey

Monitoring

- Cardiovascular:

    - ECG.

    - systemic arterial pressure.

    - central venous pressure:

        – adequate fluid replacement.

        – gauge myocardial function.

- Ventilatory:

    – rate.

    – minute volume.

    – FiO_2.

    – pulse oximetry.

    – peak airway pressure.

- Glasgow Coma Score.

- Urine output: maintain 0.5–1.0 ml kg^{-1} h^{-1}.

- Miscellaneous:

  - intracranial pressure.

  - bloods: FBC, U&E, LFT, coagulation.

Complications

- Sepsis:

  - open fractures: *Staphylococcus aureus/S. epidermidis, Escherichia coli.*

  - meningeal injury: *Streptococcus pneumoniae,* Gram –ve's.

  - GI injury: *E. coli, Bacteroides.*

  - nosocomial (30%): *Pseudomonas, Enterobacter, Klebsiella, E. coli.*

- Respiratory failure:

  - chest injury, spinal cord injury, metabolic acidosis.

  - protein leakage following endothelial injury, associated vasoconstriction: results in impaired diffusion and arterial hypoxaemia.

- Renal failure:

  - hypovolaemia, urethral damage (pelvic fracture).

  - acute tubular necrosis (ischaemia, myoglobinuria).

  - oliguria (↑ potassium, ↓ sodium) secondary to ADH release.

- Hepatic failure.

- GI stress ulceration:

  - acute GI bleed associated with sepsis and head injury.

  - incidence decreased by enteral nutrition.

- Multiple Organ Dysfunction Syndrome (see Multisystem failure and systemic inflammatory response syndrome).

Prognosis

With the widespread implementation of ATLS®, outcomes have improved in recent years.

Related subjects

Chapter 5, Scoring.

Cross-reference

Chapter 2, p. 19.   CSiG

Further reading

American College of Surgeons Committee on Trauma, *ATLS® Student Manual* (American College of Surgeons, 1997).

The New Airds Companion in Surgical Studies. Eds: Burnard KG, Young AE. Churchill Livingstone, London 1998.

BURNS

Forty thousand people are admitted to hospital in the UK every year as a result of burns. These result in 700–800 deaths per year.

Classification

The depth of the burn can either be graded as superficial or deep or alternatively the classification can be based on the 'degree' of the burn:

- First-degree burn: epidermis partially destroyed, basal membrane intact.

- Second-degree burn (superficial): basal membrane partially destroyed.

- Second-degree burn (deep): basal membrane entirely destroyed, dermis partially destroyed, epidermal cells still present around hair follicles.

- Third-degree burn: epidermis and dermis totally destroyed, subcutaneous tissue damage, in very severe cases even deeper tissues and organs affected.

An alternative classification is based on the cause:

- Physical:
  - heat.
  - electricity.
  - radiation.
- Chemical.

Causes

Burns occur when there is destruction or damage of some or all of the different layers of cells which form human skin, and on occasion the deeper tissues and organs:

- Thermal.

- Non-ionising (UV) or ionising (γ) radiation.

- Electricity.

- Chemicals.

- Respiratory injuries from smoke inhalation.

Increasing thermal exposure results in increasing tissue damage: 75°C for 1 s will cause a partial thickness burn; for 10 s will cause a full-thickness burn.

Pathophysiology

- Process caused by the transfer of thermal energy from a heat source to a part of the human body surface.

- Large amount of fluid loss from the microcirculation due to the release of vasoactive peptides from damaged tissue, resulting in increased capillary permeability. This leads to oedema.

- Heat loss from the skin.

- Increase in metabolic rate about twofold.

- Cardiac output drops due to the decrease in plasma volume.

The chain of events is illustrated in Figure 3.7.

- [1–3 h]: vasodilation → oedema

- [12–24 h]: decreased perfusion → local tissue ischaemia

- Platelet adhesion → thrombosis

- Wound repair

Figure 3.7: Pathological chain of events following a burn.

Following a burn, a number of physiological processes occur:

- Hypovolaemia secondary to increased microvascular permeability and interstitial oedema.

- 40–60% decrease in cardiac output.

- Hypoxia (hypovolaemic shock + increased O_2 consumption).

- Increased metabolic requirement.

Smoke inhalation produces its own complications:

- Airway compromise, oedema and obstruction (emergency).

- Airway irritation → bronchospasm and mucus production.

- Decreased lung compliance.

- Increased lung lymph production.

Clinical

Assess the severity of the burn by either 'the Rule of Nines' or the Lund and Browder chart (Figure 3.8). This is more accurate as it takes into account the relative differences in head, thigh and leg sizes at different ages.

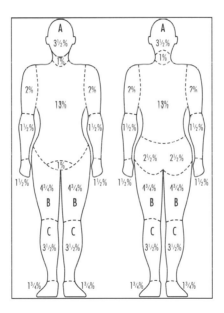

Figure 3.8: Lund and Browder chart.

Table 3.24: Relative percentages of body surface areas as affected by growth.

Age (years)	0	1	5	10	15	Adult
A – head (back or front)	9.5	8.5	6.5	5.5	4.5	3.5
B – 1 thigh (back or front)	2.75	3.25	4.0	4.25	4.5	4.75
C – 1 leg (back or front)	2.5	2.5	2.75	3.0	3.25	3.5

Smoke inhalation management is outlined in Figure 3.9.

Investigations	carboxyhaemoglobin arterial blood gases (see Chapter 2, Interpretation of special investigations) fibreoptic bronchoscopy
Treatment	intubate and 100% oxygen CPAP and PEEP regular bronchodilators chest physiotherapy

Figure 3.9: Management of smoke inhalation.

Treatment

- Resuscitation (A, B, C).

- Secure airway if evidence of an inhalational injury.

- If evidence of laryngeal oedema (cough, stridor, hoarse voice, carbon deposits around mouth) intubation by senior anaesthetist.

- IV fluid replacement is necessary for children with > 10% burns and for adults with > 15%. Fluid replacement with either colloid or crystalloid should be instigated as soon after a major burn as possible, and should be in line with one of the recommended regimens, e.g. Parkland (ATLS®):

  Weight (kg) × % burn surface area × (2–4).

- Analgesia: morphine IV (≥ 20 mg) may be necessary.

- Nutritional support for patients with extensive (> 20%) burns (see Nutrition in the critically ill) to prevent protein catabolism. The basal metabolic rate in a patient with major burns at least doubles. Nutritional requirements are:
  - adult: 20 kcal kg^{-1} + 70 kcal/% burn day^{-1}.
  - child: 60 kcal kg^{-1} + 35 kcal/% burn day^{-1}.

- Once the life has been saved attention can be turned to management of the burn itself.

- Escharotomy may be necessary for extensive chest burns to facilitate respiratory function: this can be a life-saving measure for circumferential chest burns.

- Smoke inhalation should be treated by intubation and ventilation and possibly hyperbaric oxygen where carboxyhaemoglobin > 15%. (Figure 3.9)

- Ventilatory support (see Chapter 2, Respiratory failure) may be necessary.

- Cover burns with cling film:

  - allows viewing of burns.

  - stops air flow over burns, reducing pain and heat loss.

- Transfer to a burns centre as appropriate (Table 3.25).

Table 3.25: Criteria for transfer to a burns centre.

Second- and third-degree burns > 10% TBSA in patients < 10 or > 50 years of age
Second- and third-degree burns to > 20% TBSA in all other ages
Third-degree burns > 5% TBSA in patients of any age
All second- and third-degree burns with the threat of functional or cosmetic impairment to the face, hands, feet, genitalia, perineum or major joints
All electrical burns, including lightning injuries
Chemical burns
Burns involving inhalation injury
Circumferential burns of the extremities and/or chest
Burns involving concomitant trauma among which the burn injury poses the greatest risk of morbidity or mortality.
Burns in patients with pre-existing medical conditions that may complicate management and/or prolong recovery, such as coronary artery disease, lung disease or diabetes

Monitoring

- Skin and core temperatures:

  - a decreasing skin temperature in the presence of a rising core temperature is indicative of hypovolaemia.

  - hypothermia should be avoided.

- Volume assessment:

  - urine output should be used as a monitor of perfusion, with a level of 1 ml kg^{-1} h^{-1} in children and 50 ml h^{-1} in adults as the minimum acceptable level.

  - blood pressure: only reliable as volume indicator if low.

  - pulse: young patient, < 120, reasonable perfusion; pulse > 130, increase fluid: elderly or with heart disease, pulse not accurate reflection of perfusion.

- hydration should be maintained such that the haematocrit is ~0.35.
- Arterial blood gases:
  - high risk of hypoxemia, hypercapnia due to direct pulmonary complications of burn and treatment.
  - base deficit very useful indicator of tissue oxygenation (if increasing give more fluid).
- Carboxyhaemoglobin should be monitored until in the normal range.
- Peripheral perfusion: for circumferential arm, leg burns:
  - use of Doppler to monitor.
  - if circumferential burn with decreasing pulse pressure consider escharotomy.
- Pulmonary artery occlusion pressure: for high risk patient (elderly) inhalation, cardiac output, mixed venous oxygen pressure, if cardiopulmonary stability cannot be achieved.

Complications
Fluid loss

- Occurs immediately.
- At a maximum at 2 h post-burn.
- Lasts 8–36 h.
- Plasma leakage can cause hypovolaemic shock when the burn surface area is > 15% in adults and 10% in children and infants.
- Shock as a result of severe burns is characterised by tachycardia, low central venous and arterial pressures, increased haematocrit and decreased urinary output.

Infection

- Burnt skin can no longer protect from atmospheric bacterial contamination, and great care should be exercised in the attempt to control infection by proper local treatment: this should be carried out if possible, in severe cases, in specialised treatment centres.
- Commonest organisms for infection.
  - Gram –ve organisms.
  - *Staphylococcus aureus*.
  - MRSA.
  - *Pseudomonas aeruginosa*.

- *Streptococcus pyogenes.*
- Sepsis can result in systemic inflammatory response syndrome (SIRS) (see Multisystem failure and systemic inflammatory response syndrome) and multiple organ dysfunction.
- Risk factors for infection are:
  - host factors:
    - > 30% burn surface area.
    - pre-existing disease.
    - local wound.

ARDS and multi-organ failure
Seizures

- In children especially.
- Hyponatraemia.

Renal failure

- Three major contributing factors:
  - inadequate resuscitation.
  - toxic effects of haem pigments.
  - sepsis.
- Rhabdomyolysis (see Chapter 4, Rhabdomyolysis).

Prognosis

Dependent on burn size and depth, patient age and smoke inhalation. Prevention of infection and early replacement of fluid losses remain key factors in achieving a good outcome.

Burns of > 40% BSA, age > 60 years and presence of inhalation injury are risk factors for death. The mortality rate is 0.3% with no risk factors, 3% with one, 33% with two and ~87% with three.

Cross-reference

Chapter 2, p. 47. CSiG

Cussons PD. Immediate care of the burned patient requiring hospital treatment. *Surgery* 1999; 17: 110–14. SURGERY

Freelander E. Late management of burns. *Surgery* 1999; 17: 115–19. SURGERY

Further reading

Settle JAD (ed.). *Principles and Practice of Burns Management* (Edinburgh: Churchill Livingstone, 1996).

FAT EMBOLISM SYNDROME (FES)

FES is an infrequent, potentially fatal complication of long bone fractures occurring with an incidence reported to be between 0.25 and 29%.

Definition

A clinical condition characterised by a triad of respiratory insufficiency, cerebral dysfunction and petechial haemorrhage.

Table 3.26: Gurd and Wilson's diagnostic criteria for FES.

Major	Minor	Laboratory
Petechial rash on upper anterior body	Tachycardia	Acute ↓ haemoglobin
Respiratory symptoms, signs or X-ray changes	Pyrexia	Sudden thrombocytopenia
Cerebral signs unrelated to head injury	Retinal changes	↑ ESR
	Renal changes	Fat macroglobulinaemia
	Jaundice	

From Gurd AR, Wilson RI. The Fat Embolism Syndrome *Journal of Bone and Joint Surgery* 1974; 56B: 408–16.

Diagnosis

Diagnosis is made based on the criteria of Gurd and Wilson (Table 3.26). One major and four minor criteria are required, including fat macroglobulinaemia (> 8 μm).

Causes

Closed long bone and pelvic fractures are responsible for the majority of cases of FES. Other recognised causes include:

- Acute pancreatitis.
- Burns.
- Joint reconstruction.
- Liposuction.
- Cardiopulmonary bypass.

- Total parenteral nutrition.

- Decompression sickness.

- Diabetes mellitus.

Pathophysiology

The main effect is the occlusion of small vessels in the lung by fat emboli. This results pathologically in identical lung damage to ARDS.

There are two theories to the formation of the fat emboli:

- Mechanical theory: long bone trauma leads to the release of marrow fat globules which embolise and obstruct pulmonary and systemic vessels.

- Biochemical theory; chylomicrons released at the time of trauma coalesce with very low density lipoproteins to form fat macroglobules which are toxic to pneumocytes and lead to interstitial haemorrhage, oedema and pneumonitis.

Clinical

The onset of symptoms is usually within 24 h but may take up to 72 h.

Symptoms can be divided into respiratory, central nervous system and others (Table 3.27).

Table 3.27: Signs and symptoms of FES.

Respiratory	CNS	Other
Dyspnoea	Anxiety	Petechial rash
Tachypnoea	Irritation	Retinal haemorrhages
Hypoxaemia*	Confusion	Tachycardia
CXR: bilateral infiltrates	Convulsions	Fever
ARDS	CT: cerebral oedema	

*Hypoxaemia can persist up to 14 days.

Investigations

- ABG: hypoxaemia, hypocarbia.

- FBC: ↓ haemoglobin, ↓ platelets, ↓ haematocrit.

- Biochemistry: ↑ lipase (non-specific: may be increased due to bone trauma).

- COAG: coagulopathy.

- Hypocalcaemia.

- CXR: bilateral infiltrates ('snow storm' appearance), ↑ pulmonary markings, right heart dilatation.

- ECG: ST segment ischaemic changes, right ventricular strain.

Treatment

The mainstay of treatment of FES is supportive.

- Respiratory support:

  - oxygen.

  - CPAP.

  - IPPV.

- Cardiovascular support:

  - maintain intravascular volume.

  - maintain oxygen delivery.

  - inotropes may be necessary.

- CNS: control intracranial pressure.

- Musculoskeletal: immobilise (reduce and stabilise) fracture.

Prognosis

The mortality rate of FES is ~10% usually from respiratory failure. Those who survive have an excellent prognosis. Mortality and morbidity rates can be reduced by vigilance, early diagnosis and prophylactic oxygen administration.

Cross-reference

Chapter 2, p. 46. CSiG

Further reading

Gurd AR, Wilson RI. Fat embolism syndrome. *Journal of Bone and Joint Surgery* 1974; 58: 408–16.

4

PROBLEMS IN INTENSIVE CARE

Sepsis

Localised Infections

MRSA

Nosocomial Infections

Pyrexia

Rhabdomyolysis

Brain Stem Death

SEPSIS

Definition

The development of systemic inflammatory response syndrome (SIRS) as the result of an infective process, manifested by two or more of:

- Temperature >38 or < 36°C.
- Tachycardia > 90 min^{-1}.
- Tachypnoea > 20 min^{-1} or hyperventilation to PaCO$_2$ < 4.25 kPa.
- WBC >12 × 10^9 or < 4 × 10^9.

Immunocompromised patients can be septic without eliciting an inflammatory response.

Classification

- Surgical and postoperative:
  - wound.
  - peritoneal:

    abscess.

    – peritonitis.
  - pulmonary.
  - prosthetic.
  - septicaemia.
  - pseudomembranous colitis.
- Immunocompromised.
- Organism.

Pathophysiology

Predisposing factors

- Change in microenvironment: antibiotics reduce gut-colonising flora increasing susceptibility to pathogens.
- Disruption of intestinal mediators: villous ischaemia.
- Ischaemia-reperfusion injury: mediator related (? oxygen-free radicals).
- Blood loss and transfusion: decreased efficiency of immunological and hepatic cells to clear bacteria and endotoxin.
- Malnutrition.
- Immunocompromised patients.

Microorganisms

- Cutaneous: Gram +ve cocci.
- Wound:
  - Gram +ve cocci.
  - enterococci.
  - *Escherichia coli.*
  - *Pseudomonas aeruginosa.*
- GI/urological:
  - Gram –ve.
  - *Escherichia coli.*
  - *Klebsiella.*
  - enterobacter.
  - *Proteus.*
  - MRSA (see below).

Mediators

- Pro-inflammatory
  - tumour necrosis factor (TNF).
  - interleukins 6 and 8.
  - platelet-activating factor.
- Anti-inflammatory
  - interleukins 4, 10, 11, 13.
  - transforming growth factor β.

(TNF is the principal mediator of sepsis.)

Clinical

Prevention

- Decrease bacterial count.
- Decrease contamination.
- Surgical technique.
- Environmental.
- Antibiotic prophylaxis.
- Decrease hospital stay

Investigations

- Surgical wound and swab.

- Catheter (vascular, urological and drainage).

- Chest examination and CXR.

- Urine microscopy and culture.

- Sputum culture/broncho-alveolar lavage (see Chapter 6, Broncho-alveolar lavage).

- Ultrasound for fluid collections.

Nosocomial infection has an incidence in ITU of 15–20% in non-ventilated and 18–60% in ventilated patients.

Treatment

- Recognise developing sepsis.

- Resuscitate and restore organ perfusion and oxygenation:
  - fluid resuscitation.
  - supportive measures.

- Identify primary pathology.

- Treat primary pathology:
  - antibiotics.
  - abscess drainage:
    - surgical.
    - radiological.

Complications

SIRS and MODS (see Chapter 3, Multisystem failure and systemic inflammatory response syndrome).

LOCALISED SEPSIS

Pneumonia

- Inflammatory disease of the lung.

- Associated with tissue consolidation due to alveolar flooding with proteinaceous exudate.

- Neutrophil inflammatory response → high-pressure pulmonary oedema → alveolar consolidation.

- Co-existent systemic infective signs.

- Nosocomial pneumonia is responsible for 15% of nosocomial infections (see below).

Investigations

- Blood gases: hypoxia secondary to shunting.

- Sputum microscopy: neutrophil infiltrates.

- Broncho-alveolar lavage (see below): more precise cultures.

- Chest radiograph (CXR) (Figure 4.1).

Organisms and treatment

Table 4.1 outlines the organisms commonly causing pneumonia and their treatments.

Table 4.1: Causes and treatment of pneumonia.

Patient	Organism	Treatment
Young healthy adult	*Streptococcus pneumonia* *Mycobacterium pneumonia* viral	penicillin, cephalosporin, erythromycin erythromycin, tetracycline supportive care
Elderly and diabetics	*Streptococcus pneumonia* *Legionella* *Mycobacterium tuberculosis* influenza Gram −ve bacilli	penicillin, cephalosporin, erythromycin erythromycin ≥ two of isoniazid, rifampicin, pyrazinamide, ethambutol, streptomycin supportive cephalosporin, aminoglycoside
Seizures	anaerobes (aspiration)	cephalosporin, aminoglycoside
Alcoholism	*Streptococcus pneumonia* Gram −ve bacilli (*Klebsiella*)	penicillin, cephalosporin, erythromycin cephalosporin, aminoglycoside
Chronic lung disease	*Streptococcus pneumonia* *Haemophilus influenzae* Gram −ve bacilli	penicillin, cephalosporin, erythromycin ampicillin cephalosporin, aminoglycoside
AIDS	*Pneumocystis carinii* *Streptococcus pneumonia* *Haemophilus influenzae* *Mycobacterium tuberculosis*	trimethoprim-sulphamethoxazole or pentamidine penicillin, cephalosporin, erythromycin ampicillin ≥ two of isoniazid, rifampicin, pyrazinamide, ethambutol, streptomycin

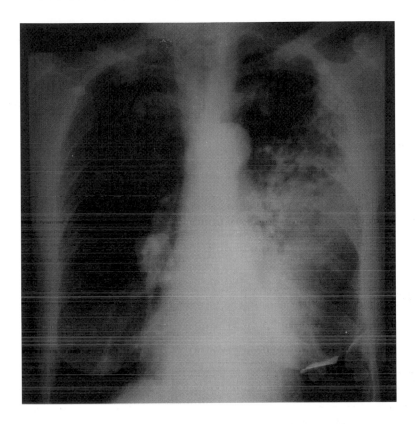

Figure 1.1: PA chest radiograph of a woman showing that she has had the chest radiograph performed with ECG leads still *in situ*. There is shadowing in the left mid- and upper zones that obscure the left heart border. Within the area of shadowing there appears to be the presence of an air bronchogram. Appearances are suggestive of consolidation in the left upper lobe. There is no evidence of any consolidation in the right lung, which appears clear. Cardiac size is within normal limits. A prominent aortic knuckle is noted. (Reproduced from Radiology Made Easy, GMM, 1999).

Lung abscess

Definition

Necrosis of lung tissue with suppuration.

Clinical

Predisposing factors:

- Aspiration of oral flora:

  - decreased level of consciousness.

  - vomiting.

- Post-pneumonic: immunocompromised, alcohol abuse, diabetic.
- Secondary to regional sepsis.

Symptoms and signs

- Malaise.
- Fever and rigors.
- Cough.
- Foul-smelling purulent sputum.
- CXR

Organisms

- Anaerobes.
- *Streptococcus*.
- *Fusobacteria*.
- *Bacteroides*.

Treatment

- Specific antibiotics (including anaerobic cover): benzyl-penicillin and metronidazole.
- Early bronchoscopy:
  - rules out stenotic lesion.
  - ensures free drainage.

Complications

- Haemoptysis.
- Pyopneumothorax: secondary to abscess rupture.
- Empyema.
- Endobronchial spread to other areas of lung.

Bronchiectasis

Definition
A condition with chronic inflammation of lobar bronchi which become dilated and chronically infected.

Aetiology

- Childhood infections: whooping cough.

- Systemic diseases: cystic fibrosis, hypogammaglobulinaemia.

Pathophysiology

- Impaired mucociliary function.

Clinical

- Persistent cough productive of purulent sputum.

- Intermittent haemoptysis.

- Frequent infective exacerbations.

The investigation of choice is a CT scan (Figure 4.2) with 3D reconstruction.

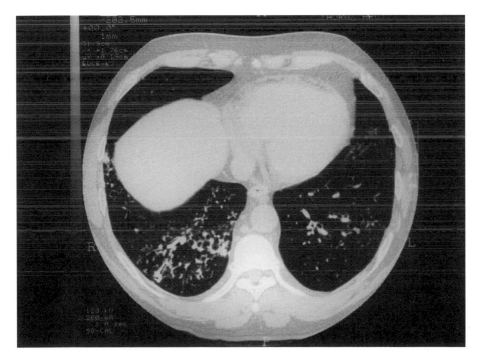

Figure 4.2: Section of a high-resolution CT scan study of the chest. The technique takes thin sections of the chest allowing a very detailed look at the lung parenchyma. Bilateral basal bronchiectasis is seen (dilated bronchi in the periphery of the lung). (Reproduced from Radiology Made Easy, GMM, 1999).

Treatment

- Keep airways free: postural drainage.

- Treat active infection.

- Surgical excision (conservative resection) of localised unilateral areas of bronchiectasis.

- Surgical high-risk patients with bronchiectasis may benefit from pre-operative optimisation on ITU (see Chapter 5, Preoperative management, optimisation and intra-operative care).

Complications

- Failure to thrive in children.

- Recurring pneumonia.

- Chronic infection, amyloid and brain abscesses are all extremely rare now.

Prognosis

The vast majority of patients lead an active life.

Empyema thoracis

Definition

Pus in the pleural cavity

Aetiology

- Effusion post-pneumonia.

- Ruptured lung abscess.

- Secondary to subphrenic abscess.

- Secondary to traumatic haemothorax (infected).

- Oesophageal perforation.

- Postoperative.

Clinical

- Most commonly bacterial.

- Complication of a more basic pathology (bacterial pneumonia).

- Diagnosis:
  - CXR.
  - thoracocentesis.

Treatment

- Adequate drainage of pus:

    - large (14 G) -bore needle thoracocentesis.

    - Chest tube (see Chapter 6, Intercostal chest tube drainage) (28–40 F).

    - Surgical:

        - mini-thoracotomy.

        - formal thoracotomy.

        - video-assisted thoracoscopic.

Complications

- Uncontrollable sepsis.

- Respiratory failure (see Chapter 2).

- Fibrothorax: restrictive ventilatory deficit.

Acute mediastinitis

Acute mediastinitis is a very dangerous condition, resulting in marked systemic disturbance and sometimes resulting in cardiovascular collapse.

Causes

- Perforation of a mediastinal viscus (oesophagus):

    - instrumentation.

    - spontaneous (Boerhaave's rupture).

- Penetrating trauma.

- Complication of (cardiac) surgery (see Chapter 1, Cardiac output: physiology and pharmacology).

Clinical signs

- Severe sepsis.

- Very marked tachycardia.

- Dysrrhythmia most commonly atrial fibrillation.

- Decreased cardiac output.

Clinical investigation

- Chest X-ray

    - mediastinal widening:

    - posterior mediastinal fluid level.

    - sympathetic pleural effusion.

Treatment

- Thoracotomy and repair of oesophageal rupture/exteriorisation of oesophagus (treating any underlying pathology: oesophageal carcinoma).

- Mediastinal drainage.

- Broad-spectrum antibiotics.

Complications

- Spread of infection:

    - empyema: via colonisation of sympathetic pleural effusion.

    - neck: ascending infection leading to laryngeal obstruction.

Urinary tract infections

Colonisation of the urinary tract is common in ITU. In 20% of cases this progresses to UTI. Of nosocomial UTI, 80% are catheter related. UTI are the most common nosocomial infection (see below).

Classification

UTI encompasses a broad spectrum of conditions (Table 4.2).

Table 4.2: Spectrum of urinary tract infections.

Adult non-specific infection	Specific infection	Special situations
Asymptomatic bacteriuria	genitourinary TB	UTI in children
Asymptomatic cystitis	fungal infections	UTI in pregnancy
Recurrent cystitis	parasitic infections	UTI in the elderly
Acute pyelonephritis	viral infections	catheter-associated UTI*
Chronic pyelonephritis		post-urological surgery*
Epididymitis		
Prostatitis		

*Most important in critical care.

Diagnosis

- MSU: avoids contamination from colonisation of distal urethra.
- Urinalysis:
  - bacteria.
  - microscopy: WBC, RBC, casts, epithelial cells.
  - pH: alkaline pH > 7: *Proteus* infection.
- Bloods: U&E: renal dysfunction secondary to Gram –ve bacteraemia.
- Ultrasound renal tract.
- Scintigraphy: renal function.
- Radiography:
  - renal damage.
  - reflux.

Pathogenesis

- Colonisation → ascending infection.
- Intra-/extraluminal migration of bacteria.

Clinical

- Fever.
- Leucocytosis.
- Bacteraemia.
- Lower abdominal and back pain.

Diagnosis

- > 10^5 cfu mm^{-3} in urine culture.
- Supported by pyuria ± haematuria.

Organisms

- Catheter-associated infections:
  - *Escherichia coli*: 30%.
  - *Enterococcus*: 15%.
  - *Pseudomonas aeruginosa*: 12.5%.
  - *Klebsiella*: 7.6%.
  - *Proteus*: 7.3%.
  - More than one organism is not uncommon.

Treatment

- Prevention:
  - avoid unnecessary catheterisations.
  - aseptic catheter insertion.
  - sterile technique to obtain specimens.
  - change catheter only if necessary.
- Remove (and replace) catheter.
- Urine culture and sensitivity.
- Empirical treatment:
  - cephalosporin/4-quinolone.
  - seek advice from microbiologist.

Complications

- Fever.
- Pyelonephritis.
- Perinephric abscess.
- Bacteraemia and sepsis.

Mortality rate

UTI are responsible for 13% of all bacteraemic deaths.

Cross reference

Buck AC. Urinary tract infection. *Surgery* 1999; 17: 145–50. SURGERY

MRSA

- Methicillin-resistant *Staphylococcus aureus*.
- Cause of numerous nosocomial infections (see below).
- Multiple resistance to antibiotics.
- Several strains.
- Responsible for serious problems in ITU.

Infections

- Nosocomial pneumonia.

- Wound infection.

- Intravascular catheter infection.

- Burns.

- Recurrent infections post-transplantation.

- Cross infection.

Treatment

- Prevention: hand washing, no sharing of thermometers and stethoscopes.

- Isolation of known carriers: theatre, wards and ITU.

- Vancomycin 1 g bd.

- Ciprofloxacin.

Cross-reference

Chapters 21, p. 221, and 20, p. 211. CSiG

Finch R. Antimicrobial therapy principles of use. *Surgery* 1999; 17: SURGERY 138–40.

NOSOCOMIAL INFECTIONS

Nosocomial infections affect 5–10% of admitted patients with an increased risk in ITU because of the frequency of invasive and multiple procedures, the presence of indwelling devices and the presence of patients with impaired immune systems (trauma, burns).

Definition

Infection that develops as a result of patient's admission.

Classification

- ITU acquired (67%).

- Hospital acquired (33%).

Clinical

Table 4.4 details organ system, risk factors, organisms and empirical treatment.

Different types of surgery influence the risk of wound infection (Table 4.4).

Management

Outbreaks require the involvement of a multidisciplinary infection control team including intensivist, surgeon, microbiologist and infection control nurse.

For an isolated case the two questions that need to be asked are:

- What is the most likely causative microorganism?
- What are the most appropriate antibiotics?

Table 4.3: Nosocomial infections, organisms and treatment.

Nosocomial infection	Incidence (%)	Risk factors	Organisms	Empirical treatment
UTI	40	catheter	Gram –ve, *Escherichia coli, Candida albicans*	remove catheter, cephalosporin, 4-quinolone
Pneumonia	15	intubation tracheotomy, ITU, recent surgery, increased age, immuno-suppressed, chronic lung disease, opiates	enterobacteria, *Klebsiella, Escherichia coli, Serratia, Pseudomonas, Staphylococcus aureus, Haemophilus, Streptococcus pneumoniae*	third-generation cephalosporin, imipenem, vancomycin if MRSA prevalent
Vascular catheter-related	8	duration > 72 h, IV catheter, skin colonisation, poor technique, site (leg > arm)	*Staphylococcus aureus, Staphylococcus epidermidis,* Gram –ve, *Candida*	flucloxacillin and gentamicin, vancomycin if MRSA prevalent
Primary blood stream infection*			Coagulase –ve, *Staphylococcus, Enterococcus, Staphylococcus aureus*	third-generation cephalosporin
Surgical wound	20	Type of surgery (see Table 4.4) Long procedure Nutrition Diabetes Chronic Renal Failure	*Staphylococcus aureus, Enterococcus, Escherichia coli,* coagulase –ve, *Staphylococcus, Pseudomonas*	

*Diagnosed by positive blood culture, clinical sepsis and no other recognised cause for infection.

Table 4.4: Surgical infection risk.

Procedure type	Infection risk (%)
Clean	< 10
Clean-contaminated	10–15
Contaminated	20
Dirty	30–40

Prognosis

- 3% of patients die from nosocomial infections.
- ITU pneumonia has a 30% mortality rate.

Further reading

Vincent J-L, Bihari DJ *et al.* The prevalence of nosocomial infections in Intensive Care Units in Europe. *Journal of the American Medical Association* 1995; 274: 639–44.

PYREXIA

Definition

The elevation of body temperature above normal (37.4°C).

Classification

Pyrexias are classified by degree of fever (Table 4.5).

Causes

The causes of pyrexia are evenly broken down into infectious and non-infectious (Figure 4.3).

Timing of postoperative pyrexias (Table 4.6)

Clinical effects of pyrexia

- Increased oxygen requirement.
- Confusion.
- Decreased BP (vasodilation).

Management

Investigations

- Wound:
  - oedema, tenderness, erythema, purulent discharge.
  - swab → M, C and S.

Table 4.5: Classification of pyrexia.

Grade	Temperature (°C)	Cause
Low	< 38.9	majority of cases are non-infectious
Intermediate	38.9–41.1	vast majority of infectious causes. Some non-infectious causes
High	> 41.1	almost always non-infectious: malignant hyperpyrexia, hypothalamic disorders, heat stroke, drug reactions

Table 4.6: Postoperative pyrexia timing.

< 48 h	atelectasis. The effect on the hypothalamus of general anaesthesia
<72 h	not usually due to infection (except gas gangrene)
> 5 days	wound infection, anastamotic breakdown, abscess

- Chest:
    - broncho-alveolar lavage (see Chapter 6).
    - chest X-ray.
- Urine: M, C and S.
- Blood:
    - blood cultures.
    - central line swabs → M, C and S.
    - central line tips → M, C and S.
- Anastomotic breakdown.
- Transfusion reaction.

Treatment

- Treat underlying cause:
    - antibiotics.
    - surgical drainage.
    - exploration of anastomosis.
- Passive cooling.
- Anti-pyretics: used since pyrexia results in increased insensible water loss. They have two detrimental effects: (1) decrease the febrile response, a body defence mechanism; and (2) eliminate the pulse/temperature relationship upon which therapeutic decisions and assessment of response are made.

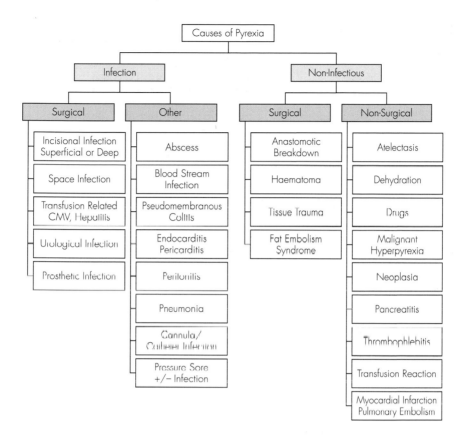

Figure 4.4: Causes of pyrexia.

Prognosis

- In the absence of infection, fever rarely persists beyond 5 days.
- Prolonged fever carries a poorer prognosis.

Further reading

Cunha BA. Fever in the intensive care unit. *Intensive Care Medicine* 1999; 25: 648–51.

RHABDOMYOLYSIS

Definition

A syndrome caused by the release of muscle cell contents (especially myoglobin) into the plasma following skeletal muscle injury.

Causes (Table 4.7)

Table 4.7: Causes of rhabdomyolysis.

Ischaemia	compression injury, compartment syndrome, vascular injury
Muscle activity/injury	seizures, burns, electric shocks, lightning, prolonged immobilisation
Drugs	alcohol, cocaine, LSD, amphetamines, lipid lowering drugs
Infection	*Escherichia coli, Salmonella*
Metabolic disease	diabetes (ketoacidosis and hyperosmolar non-ketotic)
Miscellaneous	Limb tourniquet and arterial embolism

Pathophysiology

The molecular basis for rhabdomyolysis is due to impairment of the sarcolemmic Na^+:K^+ pump. This results in:

- Decreased Na^+ extrusion.

- Decreased Ca^{2+} and H_2O efflux.

- Myofibril disruption.

- Muscle damage.

Rhabdomyolysis damages predominantly type II (red) muscle fibres, leading to myoglobin release. This results in a serum myoglobin rise, before that of the creatine kinase (CK).

Investigations

- CK/creatine phosphokinase (CPK):

    - five times upper limit of normal.

    - begins to rise 2–12 h after injury.

    - increased for several days after muscle injury (peaks at 1–3 days, declines from 3 to 5 days).

- Electrolytes: specifically:

    - hyperkalaemia: muscle necrosis leads to potassium release. Renal failure and acidosis increase this further.

- early hypocalcaemia and late hypercalcaemia. Late hypercalcaemia leads to calcium deposition in necrotic muscles.

- hyperuricaemia: due to hepatic conversion of purines released from damaged muscle.

- hyperphosphataemia: due to phosphate leakage from damaged cells.

- Arterial blood gases: metabolic acidosis.

- Urinalysis: proteinuria, haematuria and myoglobinuria.

- ↑ Urea:creatinine ratio.

- ↑ CA (carbonic anhydrase) III: more specific marker than myoglobin or CK.

- ↑ LDH (lactate dehydrogenase): non-specific.

Clinical symptoms

- Muscular: pain, weakness, tenderness, stiffness.

- Urinary: dark urine.

- Non-specific: malaise, fever, tachycardia, nausea and vomiting.

Treatment

The principal aim is to maintain an adequate circulating volume and sufficient urine output to prevent renal complications:

- Hydration:

  - large quantities of fluid to maintain urine output and adequate hydration.

  - aim for urine output > 300 ml h^{-1} until urine is myoglobin free.

  - monitor fluid balance, urine output, CVP ± PAOP.

- Reduce excessive exertion with sedatives/anticonvulsants.

- Reduce hyperthermia by controlling excessive muscle activity and passive cooling.

- Correct electrolyte imbalance:

  - hyperkalaemia: treatment of choice is insulin + glucose.

  - hyperphosphataemia: oral phosphate binding agent (calcium carbonate).

- hypocalcaemia: normally corrects with treatment of hyperphosphataemia; supplementary calcium should only be administered in tetany.

- Correct acidosis.

- Alkalinisation of urine with sodium bicarbonate to prevent dissociation of myoglobin into nephrotoxic metabolites.

- Consider diuretics to dilute nephrotoxic substances.

- Dialysis for uncontrolled hyperkalaemia, uraemic encephalopathy, acidosis or fluid overload.

Monitoring

- Electrolytes.

- Arterial blood gases.

- Electrocardiography.

Complications

- Nephrotoxicity and acute renal failure (see Chapter 3, Renal failure: diagnosis of renal failure, complications of renal failure):

  - occurs in between 10 and 30% of cases of rhabdomyolysis.

  - hypovolaemia and acidosis predispose patients with rhabdomyolysis to acute tubular necrosis.

- Elevated fascial compartment pressures:

  - results in compartment syndromes and should be treated promptly by surgical decompression.

  - more common in crush injuries.

- Acute respiratory failure (see Chapter 2).

- Disseminated intravascular coagulation (see Chapter 1).

- Metabolic acidosis.

- Cardiac arrhythmias.

Prognosis

With rapid recognition of the condition and prompt treatment (initially by hydration), the prognosis is excellent.

BRAIN STEM DEATH

Richard Downs

Definition

The irreversible loss of the capacity for consciousness, combined with the irreversible loss of the capacity to breathe despite the artificial maintenance of the circulation and gas exchange.

Causes

- Cerebral trauma: 43%.

- Intracranial haemorrhage: 42%.

- Cerebral anoxia: 8.5%.

- Primary cerebral tumour: 1.5%.

- Others: 5%, e.g. meningitis, encephalitis and cerebral abscess.

Extracranial causes of brainstem death are rare.

Criteria for brainstem death

1   The following preconditions must be met:

- patient is in an unresponsive apnoeic coma.

- patient's coma is due to irreversible structural brain damage with CT scan evidence, and the diagnosis is fully established.

- patient is ventilator-dependent for adequate gas exchange as spontaneous respiration has ceased altogether.

2   The following must be excluded:

- therapeutic drugs:

  - sedatives.

  - narcotic analgesics.

  - neuromuscular blocking agents.

- primary hypothermia (core temperature >35°C).

- metabolic abnormalities;

  - acidosis.

  - hyper/hyponatraemia.

- endocrine abnormalities:
    - hypothyroidism.
    - diabetic coma.
- intoxication:
    - alcohol.
    - drugs.

Diagnosis

- A series of tests confirms that all brainstem reflexes are absent.

- Performed by at least two medical practitioners, clinically independent of each other and who are > 5 years post-registration (one has to be a consultant).

- Neither practitioner must be a member of the transplant team.

- The practitioners carry out two sets of tests either separately or together and not within 6 h of the onset of coma. The tests are repeated after an unspecified interval to remove the risk of observer error.

- The legal time of death is when the first set of tests indicates brainstem death, although death is not pronounced until completion of the second set of tests.

Brainstem death tests

1 Pupils are fixed and do not respond to sharp changes in the intensity of incident light.

2 There is no corneal reflex with care being taken not to damage the cornea.

3 There are no vestibulo-ocular reflexes. Determined by absent eye movements when 50 ml ice cold water is injected over 1 min into each external auditory meatus in turn. The tympanic membrane must first be directly inspected to confirm that the external auditory meatus is not blocked.

4 There are no motor responses within the cranial nerve distribution. Tested by applying supra-orbital pressure and observing for facial and limb movements.

5 There is no gag reflex or reflex response to tracheal stimulation from a suction catheter passed into the trachea.

6   There is no respiratory effort when the respiratory centre is stimulated. This is done by administering 6 l min^{-1} O_2 via the trachea when the patient is disconnected from the ventilator and allowing the $PaCO_2$ to rise > 6.65 kPa (confirmed by arterial blood gas analysis) while observing for spontaneous respiratory effort. This must be adjusted for patients with chronic lung disease who are known to retain CO_2.

Although EEG, cerebral angiography and oesophageal contractility testing are carried out in some centres they are not required by law in the UK to make a diagnosis of brainstem death.

Why diagnose brainstem death?

- To clarify the situation for relatives and, therefore, avoid an unnecessary and distressing vigil.

- To enable decisions about further management to be taken:

  - continue care until the heart stops which is usually within a few days.

  - to remove the patient from the ventilator before the heart stops.

  - to allow the patient to become a possible organ donor.

- To prevent further nursing of a corpse.

- To enable precious ITU resources to be used to benefit other potentially salvageable patients.

Brainstem death in children

- Children > 2 months of age should be treated the same as adults.

- In premature babies the criteria for brainstem death cannot be applied.

- Between 37 weeks gestation and 2 months it is not possible confidently to diagnose brainstem death.

- Organs for transplantation may be removed from anencephalic infants when two doctors agree that spontaneous respiration has ceased.

Cross-reference

Smith M. Brain stem death. *Surgery* 1998; 16: 25–7.

Smith M. Brain stem death. *Surgery* 1999; 17: 205–7.

5

PRINCIPLES OF ICU

Indications for Admission

Preoperative Management, Optimisation and Intra-Operative Care

Organisation and Staffing

Scoring and Outcome Measures

Costs

Analgesia and Anaesthesia

Monitoring

ICU ADMISSION

ICU is a scarce resource in the UK. Therefore, ICU facilities must be prioritised based on patient need and benefit. There are several identifiable groups of patients vying for admission to the ICU:

- Patients who were previously well, but have an acute disturbance of physiology due to a potentially reversible cause, e.g. meningococcal sepsis.

- Patients with pre-existing morbidity in one or more organ systems who have an acute disturbance of physiology due to a potentially reversible cause, e.g. pneumonia, leading to respiratory failure in a patient with COAD.

- Patients who have an acute disturbance of physiology due to a cause which they are unlikely to survive, despite maximal therapy, e.g. uncontrollable massive bleeding post-RTA or severe head injury.

- Patients who are currently stable but have a disease process which may require Intensive Care in the near future. This group may warrant admission before their condition deteriorates or they get any complications, e.g. acute pancreatitis.

The ability of an ICU to accept a patient will depend on the availability of beds (this includes the provision of appropriately trained medical and nursing staff, and does not just apply to a physical bed). If the ICU is full then it may be possible to:

- Discharge an ICU patient to the ward (provided that they meet discharge criteria).

- Transfer an ICU patient to another ICU (this depends on the current condition of the patient, the local availability of ICU beds and having appropriately trained medical and nursing staff).

- Transfer the new patient to another ICU (the same problems apply).

- Care for the new patient in another area of the hospital (this cannot be recommended, except as a holding measure until a suitable location has been found for definitive care).

Referral to the ICU
- Should be made as early in the course of the disease process as possible while there remains the possibility of avoiding or reversing organ damage.

- Should ideally be made by the referring consultant to the ICU consultant.

- Should be medically appropriate (patients who are too well or too sick use valuable resources which may be better spent with greater benefit on others).

- Should comply with the wishes of the patient and their family.

Admission criteria

It is difficult to adhere to strict criteria as each case is complex and has its own merits and faults. However, there are some general points to take into consideration:

- Underlying diagnosis and severity of the current disease process.

- Degree of organ dysfunction and extent of physiological abnormalities (this may be worsened by delayed referral).

- Physiological reserve of the patient (this will be decreased by advancing age and co-existing premorbid pathology).

There are some instances where ICU admission is mandatory:

1 Mechanical or assisted ventilation for acute respiratory failure.

2 Specialised invasive monitoring, e.g. arterial line or pulmonary artery catheter.

3 Specialised treatments, e.g. haemofiltration for acute renal failure.

4 Drug infusions, e.g. inotropes or sedatives.

Discharge from the ICU

Patients may be discharged from the ICU:

- When they have fully recovered from their precipitating illness.

- When they are nearing recovery from the precipitating illness and care in an HDU is appropriate. This relies on a properly staffed HDU facility, which bridges the gap in skills between the ICU and the general wards. At present only ~15% of hospitals in the UK have an HDU.

- When they have reached a preset limit on treatment without success. This should be decided at admission and subsequently at regular intervals by the admitting and referring consultants, and discussed with the patient and family. Patients with malignancy or end-stage organ failure may be in this category.

- When there is brain stem death.

- When there is persistent vegetative state.

Discharge criteria

Although each patient should be considered individually, the following principles may be applied:

General

- Successfully treated patients with improving pathophysiology.

- No requirement for invasive monitoring, e.g. arterial line.

- No requirement for sedative or inotropic drug infusions.

- No requirement for specialist therapies, e.g. haemofiltration (unless there is a renal unit available).

Organ systems

- Respiratory:

    - can maintain and protect airway ($\pm$ tracheostomy).

    - no requirement for mechanical ventilation (for > 12 h without signs of impending respiratory failure).

    - no hypoxia (PaO_2 > 8 kPa on FiO_2 < 0.4).

    - no hypercapnoea (this will depend on the patient's normal $PaCO_2$).

- CVS:

    - haemodynamically stable.

    - no requirement for inotropic support.

- Renal:

    - adequate urine output (> 0.5 ml kg^{-1} min^{-1}).

    - planned renal support if CRF.

- Haematological:

    - stable Hb (ideally > 10 g dl^{-1}).

    - no coagulopathy.

PREOPERATIVE MANAGEMENT, OPTIMISATION AND INTRA-OPERATIVE CARE

Most patients can be anaesthetised. The challenge is to improve the patient's condition preoperatively to maximise the chances of a good outcome. Poor preparation for surgery may well result in a poor outcome. Early anaesthetic involvement in patient management is advised.

Preoperative assessment

- Previous anaesthetics:
  - difficult intubation.
  - anaphylaxis.
  - malignant hyperpyrexia.
  - suxamethonium apnoea.
  - porphyria.
  - sickle cell disease.
  - halothane toxicity.
- Coexisting disease.
- Drug interactions and reactions.
- Risk factors for infection.
- Systems assessment:
  - cardiovascular:
    - assess and optimise blood pressure control.
    - assess associated pathologies.
  - respiratory:
    - assess airway obstruction (FEV_1).
    - assess dyspnoea.
    - decrease potential postoperative complications: bronchodilators, physiotherapy, cease smoking.
  - hydration and nutrition.
- Assess airway: ? potential difficult intubation.
- ASA status (Table 5.1).

Table 5.1: American Society of Anaesthesiologists physical status classification.

I	Healthy patient
II	Mild systemic disease with no functional limitation
III	Severe systemic disease with functional limitation
IV	Severe systemic disease that is a constant threat to life
V	Moribund patient not expected to live 24 h with or without surgery

E, emergency.

Optimisation

The term 'optimisation' refers to the improvement of the patient's condition before surgery. In an emergency situation optimisation may occur 'on the run'. Even a few hours on ITU can in some cases improve outcome significantly. For an elective procedure optimisation may take several weeks. Examples of optimisation efforts are outlined in Table 5.2.

Table 5.2: Some techniques of optimisation.

System	Condition	Optimisation techniques
Haematology	anaemia: chronic, acute	investigate and treat cause, transfuse
	polycythaemia	venesection and haemodilution
	sickle cell disease	oxygenate, exchange transfusion
Cardiovascular	hypertension	optimal blood pressure control
	arrhythmias	anti-arrhythmia
Respiratory	upper respiratory tract infection	delay elective procedure
	COAD	stop smoking, treat active infection: antibiotics and physiotherapy
Liver disease	hypo-albuminaemia	replacement therapy
	coagulation factor deficiency	replacement therapy

Intra-operative care

- Airway:
  - face mask.
  - laryngeal mask airway.
  - cuffed endotracheal tube.
  - surgical airway.

Only a cuffed endotracheal tube or a surgical airway offer protection against aspiration of vomit.

- Breathing:
  - spontaneous ventilation.
  - controlled ventilation (automatic ventilator/anaesthetist controlled).
- Fluids:
  - deficit: estimate initial deficit. For adults: 8 h starved = ~1000 ml.
  - maintenance: 50–150 ml h^{-1} (for adults).
  - losses: replace like with like.
- Monitoring:
  - pulse oximetry.
  - expired CO_2.
  - electrocardiogram.
  - blood pressure:
    - non-invasive.
    - intra-arterial.
  - CVP.
  - pulmonary artery occlusion pressure (PAOP).

In 1999, the American Society of Anaesthesiologists released new guidelines on minimum acceptable standards of monitoring during anaesthesia (Table 5.3). The standards are only the minimum. Additional monitoring such as CVP, PAOP and intra-arterial blood pressure will be appropriate for more complex procedures and higher risk patients.

Intra-operative and postoperative complications

Even in the best hands, complications can occur. Those most common during anaesthesia are:

- Inadequate depth of anaesthesia.
- Inadequate oxygenation.
- Cardiac problems:
  - arrhythmias.
  - hypertension.

Table 5.3: ASA Minimum Standards of Monitoring for Anaesthesia (modified).

	Standard	Monitoring
1	Qualified anaesthesia personnel shall be present in the room throughout the conduct of all general anaesthetics, regional anaesthetics and monitored anaesthesia care	
2	During all anaesthetics, the patient's oxygenation should be continually evaluated	FiO_2 measurement, pulse oximeter
3	During all anaesthetics, the patient's ventilation should be continually evaluated	clinical assessment, end-tidal CO_2 analysis, alarmed ventilator
4	During all anaesthetics, the patient's circulation should be continually evaluated	continuous ECG, HR and BP at least every 5 min, clinical: palpate pulse, auscultate heart (intra-arterial BP or oximetry)
5	During all anaesthetics, the patient's temperature should be continually evaluated	

- Blood loss.
- Temperature:
    - hypothermia.
    - malignant hyperpyrexia – stop anaesthetic, O_2, cool, dantrolene.
- Pressure areas: damage.
- Drug reactions and interactions.

Complications occurring in the immediate postoperative period are:

- Delayed recovery.
- Respiratory:
    - upper airway obstruction.
    - atelectasis→hypexia.
    - hypoventilation.
- Cardiovascular:
    - hypotension.
    - arrhythmias.

- Vascular:
  - phlebitis.
  - thrombosis.
- Renal dysfunction: oliguria and ARF.
- Hepatic dysfunction.

Cross-reference

Chapter 16, p. 171   `CSiG`

Roe PG. Perioperative fluid management. *Surgery* 1998; 16: 165–8.   `SURGERY`

Milner Q, Roe P. Perioperative Management: Anaemia. *Surgery* 1999; 17: 102–5.   `SURGERY`

Stoker MR. Care and monitoring of the anaesthetised patient. *Surgery* 1999; 17: 245–7.   `SURGERY`

Summors AC. Fit for anaesthesia. *Surgery* 1999; 17: 56–9.   `SURGERY`

STAFFING AND ORGANISATION IN THE ICU

The ICU is a team, which consists of:

- Medical staff:
  - clinical (ICU doctors and referring teams).
  - laboratory (microbiologists, haematologists and biochemists).
  - radiologists.
- Nursing staff.
- Physiotherapists.
- Dieticians.
- Pharmacists.
- Technicians.
- Radiographers.
- Management and administration staff.
- Receptionists.

Medical staff

The Intensive Care Society recommends:

- That there is consultant cover for the ICU at all times. This represents 15 sessions (each of 3.5 h) per week, for an ICU of up to 10 beds.

- These sessions will ideally be shared between three or more intensivists, one of whom is the clinical director.

- It is also recommended that these consultants maintain a clinical interest in their base speciality, usually anaesthesia or medicine.

- There should be resident cover on the ICU at all times. This is provided by SHOs or SpRs, usually from acute specialities, such as:

  - anaesthesia.

  - medicine.

  - surgery.

  - A&E.

The role of the intensivist is to coordinate the manpower and technical resources available. They will be ultimately responsible for the timing and selection of patients for admission, discharge and transfer from the ICU. They must ensure that the ICU has adequate medical cover at all times.

Nursing staff

- There should be one nurse for every patient on the ICU. This requires 6.5 nurses per bed.

- There should be two trained nurses to every untrained nurse.

- The nurse in charge should not be caring for a patient, to allow time to help with emergencies, if needed.

- Extra nurses may be required when the nursing dependency increases, e.g. for haemodynamically unstable patients or those requiring specialist therapy, such as haemofiltration.

Risk management

Intensive care is a high-risk area for negligence litigation, due to the increased incidences of morbidity and mortality. These may be minimised by:

- Ensuring that medical, nursing and other staff are screened before commencing their employment. This is sometimes difficult as locum doctors and agency nurses are often needed at short notice because of crises in staffing, but safety checks should still be carried out.

- Aim for retention of current staff and recruitment of well-trained and qualified applicants for permanent posts in the future.

- Continuing education with regular teaching and sufficient time for courses and study leave to gain or refresh skills and knowledge.

- Ensuring that the staff has frequent rest periods and that help and advice is close at hand.

The ICU can be a stressful place in which to work. This can be reduced by ensuring that each member of staff has the opportunity to talk about problems or issues that worry them. Socialising outside work can improve staff morale and promote a more pleasant working environment.

Cross-reference

Schmulian C. Organisation of critical care. *Surgery* 1998; 16: 73–7. SURGERY

SCORING SYSTEMS IN THE ICU

The principal aim of intensive care is to provide the highest level and best quality of care available to its patients. This will involve evaluating the outcome after ICU treatment, which is difficult for this group of patients. The most frequently used determinant of successful treatment is the hospital mortality rate (which is the death rate before discharge from hospital of ICU patients). This does not take into account the quality of life thereafter for the patient or their family.

The aim of scoring systems used clinically is to evaluate outcome for different groups of ICU patients. These may be used to:

- Determine different patient groups according to their severity of illness.

- Attach risk to each different group:

  - for mortality rate (survivability).

  - for division into separate groups for clinical trials.

- Compare different ICUs in different hospitals.

These scoring systems do not predict outcome or guide treatment planning for individual patients.

Problems with scoring systems:

- Risk adjustment takes into account the differences between patients that affect their risk of any particular outcome, which is independent of the care that they receive.

- Risk is increased by:

  - increasing age.

  - significant premorbid illness.

  - admitting diagnosis.

  - severity of the presenting illness.

  - emergency surgery.

These factors constitute the case mix, and case mix adjustment is the process of accounting for these in the determination and comparison of any outcome measure (usually the hospital mortality rate).

- Selection bias is an error in the predictive power if the database population differs from the sample population i.e. it has to be validated for that population.

- Lead-time bias is the effect of treatment (including treatment duration) on the patient before entering the ICU.

- There needs to be a complete and accurate data set to prevent errors from multiplying.

The commonly used ICU scoring systems are:

- APACHE. acute physiology and chronic health evaluation.

- SAPS. simplified acute physiology score.

- MPM: mortality probability models.

These systems assign different scores (weighting) to the measured variables (Table 5.4).

Scores may not only be applied to assess severity of illness, but also to severity of traumatic injury sustained. Those commonly used include the Revised Trauma Score, Abbreviated Injury Score and Injury Severity Scale.

Revised Trauma Score (RTS) (Table 5.5)

RTS correlates well with survival. RTS = 12 is associated with 99.5% survival, RTS = 6 has 63% survival and RTS = 0, 3.7% survival.

Table 5.4: Determinants of APACHE, SAPS and MPM scores.

	APACHE II	APACHE III	SAPS II	MPM II$_0$	MPM II$_{24,48,72}$
Age	1	1	1		1
Temperature	1	1	1		
Blood pressure	1	1	1	1	
Heart rate	1	1	1	1	
Respiratory rate	1	1			
Oxygenation	1	1	1		1
Arterial pH	1	2			
Serum HCO$_3^-$	1		1		
Serum Na$^+$	1	1	1		
Serum K$^+$	1		1		
Serum creatinine	1	1			1
Haematocrit	1	1			
WCC	1	1	1		
Glasgow Coma Scale	1	1	1	1	1
Urine output		1	1		1
Serum urea		1	1		
Serum albumin		1			
Serum bilirubin		1	1		
Serum glucose		1			
Mechanical ventilation		1	1	1	1
Prothrombin time					1
Vasoactive drugs					1
Past medical history	1	1	4	3	2
Surgical status	1		1	1	1
Reason for ICU admission	1	1		6	2
Source of ICU admission		1			
Status at hospital discharge	1	1	1	1	1
Total	**17**	**23**	**17**	**15**	**14**

Table 5.5: Revised trauma score.

Score	Glasgow Coma Score	Systolic blood pressure	Respiratory rate
0	3	0	0
1	4–5	1–49	1–5
2	6–8	50–75	6–9
3	9–12	76–89	> 29
4	13–15	> 89	10–29

Table 5.6: Examples of injuries in categories of the Injury Severity Scale.

AIS	1 (minor)	2 (moderate)	3 (severe, not life-threatening)	4 (severe, life threatening)	5 (critical)
External	abrasion, laceration	major abrasion	2° or 3° burn, 16–25% BSA	2° or 3° burn, 26–35% BSA	2° or 3° burn > 35% BSA
Head	awake, conjunctival abrasion	LOC < 15 min, maxilla #	LOC 15–59 min, basal skull #, vault #	LOC 15–59 min, + neurodef-icit, open # vault	unconscious, brain stent haemorrhage
Neck	pharynx contusion	oesophagus contusion	trachea crush	trachea laceration	trachea rupture
Thorax	rib #	rib open #, sternum #	lung contusion, sternum open #	myocardial contusion	aortic laceration, or rupture
Abdomen and Pelvic Contents	laceration, scrotum rupture	stomach contusion, deep laceration	bladder perforation, scrotum avulsion	bladder avulsion, splenic rupture, ovary rupture, uterus rupture	biliary tree injury, uterus rupture (2nd 3rd trimester)
Spine	acute strain	# spinous or transverse process	cord contusion, disc herniation, # body	cord lesion (incomplete)	Cord lesion (complete)
Extremities and Bony Pelvis	contusion finger/toe #	joint laceration, # (except femur)	crush injury, femur #, open #	pelvis crush, amputation	

Abbreviated Injury Score (AIS) and Injury Severity Scale (ISS) (Table 5.6).

AIS is calculated as the sum of the squares of the three highest categories from the ISS. From AIS, LD_{50} (lethal dose in 50%) has been calculated as:

- 40 (ages 15–44 years).

- 29 (ages 45–64 years).

- 20 (age > 65 years).

Cross-reference

Chapters 2, p. 49, and 37, p. 354. CSiG

Further reading

Champion *et al. Journal of Trauma* 1989; 29; 623–9.

COST OF INTENSIVE CARE

Intensive care is an expensive commodity in healthcare. Ten percent of all hospital costs are spent on the provision of intensive care. An ICU bed costs five times as much as a general ward bed. It is important to estimate the expenditure of an ICU as accurately as possible for several reasons:

- To negotiate funds for future budget allocation.

- To charge users of the unit in order to recoup costs.

- To estimate future projections for service provision, and the purchase and maintenance of equipment.

There are several factors that contribute to the costs of running an ICU:

- Fixed costs: capital costs independent of patient expenditure, e.g. rolling programmes for equipment replacement.

- Semi-fixed costs: staff costs account for the largest single component of the expenditure of the unit (~50%).

- Variable costs: drug, equipment and investigation costs per individual patient these will vary depending on:

    - intensity of care needed.

    - length of stay.

    - admitting diagnosis, with the highest costs involving:

        - renal failure and replacement.

        - sepsis.

        - pneumonia.

        - MOF.

        - vascular surgery.

    - outcome (↑ costs with poor outcome). Forty percent of hospital costs are spent on patients who die within three months of discharge from the ICU. The most expensive patient groups are those survivors who are expected to die and non-survivors who are expected to live.

Methods of costing

- Averages:

    - simple and cheap.

    - used to estimate future budgetary requirements.

- Cost banding:

  - minor, standard and complex bands.

  - each band has a daily rate based on resource consumption.

- Diagnosis:

  - requires a predictable reproducible clinical course.

  - used with single organ treatment, e.g. cardiac and neurosurgery.

- Pathophysiology, e.g. APACHE II: good for first day but poor correlation thereafter between physiological derangement and cost.

- Intervention scoring, e.g. TISS, NDSS: accurate but time-consuming.

There is little information on cost and outcome, since survival out of hospital and quality of life are difficult to quantify.

Further reading

Miranda DR, Gyldmark M. Evaluation and understanding the costs in the ICU. In *Current Practice in Critical Illness* (London: Chapman & Hall, 1996), 129–49.

Mostafa SM. The cost of ICU. *Care of the Critically Ill* 1995; 11: 28–31.

ANALGESIA AND ANAESTHESIA

- All of these drugs (Table 5.7) are respiratory depressants and appropriate equipment for the provision of assisted ventilation should always be available when they are used.

- Propofol (1–6 mg kg^{-1} h^{-1}) and midazolam (0.03–0.2 mg kg^{-1} h^{-1}) are the only two sedative agents commonly used as maintenance infusions, but midazolam levels can accumulate in patients with co-existing renal or hepatic impairment.

- Thiopentone is occasionally used for maintenance infusion in brain damaged neurosurgical patients, to decrease the cerebral metabolic demand for oxygen. This requires careful monitoring with EEG, and can lead to prolonged coma due to the accumulation of thiopentone.

- Propofol and thiopentone (and to a lesser degree etomidate) give a clear end-point for unconsciousness, and are, therefore, more suitable for use in a rapid sequence induction (RSI) technique than ketamine or midazolam.

Table 5.7: Anaesthetic and sedative drugs used in the ICU.

Drug	Induction dose (mg/kg)	Onset time (min)	Duration of action after bolus (min)	Advantages	Disadvantages	Indications
Propofol	1–2	<1	2–3	Smooth induction Minimal accumulation Rapid onset	pain on injection Hypotension	Standard induction agent Maintenance of sedation in the ICU
Thiopentone	3–5	<1	5–7	Smooth induction, Anti-convulsant	hypotension Histamine release Accumulation of metabolites	Standard induction agent (epileptic patients)
Etomidate	0.3	1–2	6–10	CVS stability	Nausea & Vomiting Pain on injection ↓ cortisol synthesis	Induction agent of choice for patients with cardiovascular risk factors
Ketamine	2 (IV), 10 (IM)	<1, 10	5–10, 12–25	CVS stability (↑ HR + BP), Can be given IM	Nausea & vomiting Hallucinogenic ↑ myocardial O_2 requirement	Induction agent of choice for field anaesthesia or shocked poorly resuscitated patients
Midazolam	0.03–0.2	3–5	60–120	Anti-convulsant	Long duration of action Gradual loss of consciousness	↓ requirements for other agents (co-induction)

Table 5.8: Opioid analgesia used in the ICU.

Drug	Bolus dose	Infusion rate	Indications	Side-effects
Morphine	2.5–5 mg	1–10 mg h^{-1}	standard regimen	pruritis, histamine release, vasodilatation →↓ BP
Fentanyl	50–100 μg	50–250 μg h^{-1}	analgesia for periods of medium duration, e.g. postoperative patients for overnight ventilation	profound respiratory depression, bradycardia, chest wall stiffness
Alfentanil	500 μg	25–50 μg min^{-1}	to cover painful stimuli of short duration, e.g. chest drain insertion, tracheostomy	requirement for assisted ventilation

Table 5.9: Muscle relaxants used in the ICU.

Drug	Bolus dose (mg kg^{-1}	Onset	Duration of action (min)	Metabolism
Suxamethonium	1–1.5	30 s	5	plasma cholinesterase
Atracurium	0.5	1.5–2 min	15–25*	liver + Hoffman degradation
Vecuronium	0.1	2–2.5 min	20–30*	liver
Rocuronium	0.9	45–60 s	40–50*	liver

*Times can be shortened by antagonism with neostigmine (anticholinesterase).

Suxamethonium has a number of side-effects including:

- ↑ K$^+$ – particularly in patients with renal failure, spinal injuries and burns.
- Myalgia.
- Precipitation of malignant hyperpyrexia.
- ↑ IOP.
- ↑ ICP.
- Some patients have a genetic deficit of plasma cholinesterase leading to prolonged effects (suxamethonium apnoea).

MONITORING

The level of monitoring required will depend on the clinical state of the patient.

Cardiovascular

- Pulse.
- Pulse oximeter.
- CVP.
- Arterial blood pressure.
- PA catheter (mixed venous gas).
- ECG: continuous display and 12-lead if any change.
- Cardiac enzymes.

Respiratory

- ABG.
- Ventilator readings: V_t, RR, PA_wP, F_iO_2, MV, PEEP, pulmonary compliance.
- SaO_2.
- $ETCO_2$.
- CXR.

Neurological

- ICP monitor.
- EEG.
- Jugular venous catheter.

Renal

- U&E, creatinine.
- Creatinine clearance.
- Urine and plasma osmolarity.
- Urine output (hourly).

Hepatic

- LFT.
- Clotting (INR).

Haematological

- FBC, differential and film.
- Clotting and platelet count.
- COP.
- CRP.

Metabolic

- Calcium.
- Phosphate.
- Magnesium.
- Short Synacthen test.
- Thyroid function tests.
- Glucose.

Clinical

Full 'top to toe' examination (at least daily).

Cross-reference

Schmulian C. Monitoring and inotropes in the ICU. *Surgery* 1998; 16: 78–83.

SURGERY

6

PRACTICAL PROCEDURES

Vascular Access

Tracheostomy

Intercostal Chest Tube Drainage

Broncho-alveolar Lavage

Diagnostic Peritoneal Lavage

Intracranial Pressure Monitoring

Pericardial Aspiration

Intra-abdominal Pressure Monitoring

VASCULAR ACCESS

Central venous lines

Indications

- Fluid infusion.

- Drug infusions (especially inotropes).

- Blood sampling.

- PA catheter insertion.

- TPN.

- Haemofiltration.

- Transvenous cardiac pacing.

Complications

- Pneumothorax/haemothorax (more common with subclavian or low internal jugular approaches).

- Arterial puncture (can be catastrophic with subclavian artery rupture since there is no way to occlude this vessel).

- Nerve injury:

    - phrenic, vagus and sympathetic chain in the neck.

    - femoral nerve in the groin.

- Cardiac arrhythmias.

- Air embolus with neck cannulation in hypovolaemic patients.

- Erosion through vessel wall (including myocardium).

- Formation of A-V fistula.

- Thoracic duct injury in the neck (with left sided cannulation).

- Infection:

    - use careful aseptic technique for insertion.

    - avoid sites with skin erythema.

    - TPN increases the risk of infection and should be infused via a dedicated line.

    - sites should be changed regularly (every 5–7 days).

- Ectopic placement:

  - ensure that free aspiration of blood is possible.

  - check position with CXR.

Contraindications to insertion

- Bleeding diatheses (especially with the subclavian route, since occlusion of a bleeding vessel is more difficult).

- Localised infection.

These are relative and clinical need must be considered for each individual case.

Internal jugular vein (IJV)
Anatomy

- IJV is formed from the jugular bulb, which drains blood from the brain via the sigmoid sinus.

- It passes through the jugular foramen and then follows a straight line to the sternoclavicular joint, where it joins the subclavian vein to form the brachiocephalic vein.

- IJV is intimately associated with the internal carotid artery throughout its course: initially posterior and finally anterolateral to it.

- IJV, internal carotid artery and vagus nerve all travel within the carotid sheath.

- IJV is superficial in the upper part of its course, covered by the sternomastoid muscle in the middle part and splits the sternal and clavicular heads of that muscle in the lower part.

Cannulation technique

1 Head down position.

2 Clean skin.

3 Infiltrate with local anaesthetic.

4 A syringe should be attached to the needle at all times to reduce the risk of pneumothorax:

   - mid/high approach: lateral to carotid artery at the level of the cricoid cartilage.

   - low approach: between the heads of sternomastoid (reduced risk of arterial puncture but increased risk of pneumothorax).

5   Insert the needle, and advance aiming towards the ipsilateral nipple.

6   Once blood is aspirated continue as in the Seldinger technique.

Seldinger technique

1   Needle with syringe attached.

2   Once blood is freely aspirated, detach the syringe and feed the guide wire (with the flexible J tip first) for ~15 cm.

3   Remove the needle (taking care not to displace wire).

4   Extend the skin incision with a scalpel blade.

5   Advance the dilator over the wire (and remove).

6   Insert the catheter over the wire.

7   Remove the wire.

8   Aspirate blood and flush all lines with heparinised saline.

9   CXR to confirm position.

Subclavian vein

Anatomy

- Continuation of the axillary vein.

- Runs from the lateral border of the first rib, and arches upwards over the rib.

- Its most cephalad point is at the mid-clavicular line.

- Joins the IJV to form the brachiocephalic vein behind the sternoclavicular joint.

- External jugular vein drains into SCV.

Cannulation technique

1   Head down position.

2   Clean skin.

3   Local anaesthetic infiltration.

4   A syringe should be attached to the needle at all times to reduce the risk of pneumothorax.

5   Needle is inserted at the mid-clavicular line or junction of medial third and lateral two thirds of clavicle.

6 'Walk-off' the clavicle aiming towards the suprasternal notch.

7 Once blood is aspirated continue as in the Seldinger technique.

Pulmonary artery flotation catheter
Insertion

- A sterile procedure: the operator should be gowned.

- Balloon is inflated for insertion and deflated for withdrawal.

- Catheter is threaded slowly (1 cm s⁻¹) by the operator via an introducer in a central vein and 'floats' on the column of blood.

- Figure 1.4 shows the pressure waves observed on correct placement.

Complications

- Entanglement of the catheter (the so-called 'knotted swan'): this may require surgical removal.

- Pulmonary infarction.

- Valve rupture.

- Ectopic placement.

- Erosion through a vessel wall (including cardiac chamber).

- Catheter is long and narrow, hence it is easily occluded.

- Arrhythmias (usually on insertion or manipulation).

Cross-reference

Chapter 37, p. 357. **CSiG**

Arterial lines

Arterial catheters

- Venflon type (cannula over needle).

- Seldinger type (wire through needle).

They are usually made out of Teflon®, which is durable and reduces thrombosis formation.

- Sites:

  - radial.

  - brachial (not good in conscious patients: because of arm bending).

- femoral.
- dorsalis pedis.
- Sizes:
    - 18 G (femoral).
    - 20 G (standard).
    - 22 G (paediatric).

Insertion technique

1 Clean skin.

2 Local anaesthetic.

3 Nick skin with hypodermic needle.

4 Angle at ~45° to skin.

5 Flush of arterial blood rises up the hub of the cannula.

6 Reduce angle to ~15–20° and cannulate artery.

Complications

- False aneurysm formation.
- Thrombosis.
- Infection (usually localised infection).
- Damped trace (low reading systolic BP, but MAP usually accurate).
- Kinking/occlusion of the catheter.
- Disconnection (risk of haemorrhage).
- Compromised blood flow distal to the catheter (this is mainly a problem for end arteries, e.g. dorsalis pedis).
- Haematoma.
- A-V fistula.
- Air embolus.
- Drugs or infusions given in error: this may be minimised by accurate labelling of the catheter.

Venous cut-down

Venous cut-down is principally used in the trauma situation. It may also be used when central venous access is impossible. Any large vein is suitable although the long saphenous vein at the ankle is the favoured site and as such will be discussed here.

Indications

- Emergency vascular access:
    - multiple trauma.
    - hypovolaemic shock.

Procedure

Any large vein, most commonly:

- Lower limb: long saphenous vein at ankle.
- Upper limb:
    - cephalic vein in forearm or arm.
    - antecubital fossa.

The technique is similar for all sites. That for the long saphenous vein will be described:

1 Transverse skin incision 2 cm anterior and superior to the medial malleolus.

2 Dissect the vein free by blunt dissection.

3 Place two ties around the vein, the distal one secured tightly, the proximal loose.

4 Perform a venotomy.

5 Insert a large 14 G cannula into the venotomy.

6 Flush the cannula with 0.9% NaCl.

7 Secure the cannula by tightening the upper ligature.

Complications

- Incorrect identification of the vein.
- Extravasation.
- Infection: infection rate may be reduced by leaving the cannula in place for < 24 h.

Further reading

Soni N. *Practical Procedures in Anaesthesia and Intensive Care* (Oxford: Butterworth-Heinemann, 1989).

Hillier JE, Brett S. Techniques of vascular access. *Surgery* SURGERY
2000; 18: 56a–c.

TRACHEOSTOMY

Indications

- Airway obstruction:
    - trauma:
        - severe maxillofacial trauma.
        - severe head injury.
        - severe facial burns.
    - infection: acute epiglottitis.
    - oedema.
- Protection of the tracheobronchial tree:
    - airway control after major oropharyngeal surgery.
    - supraglottic surgery.
    - head injury.
- Ventilatory insufficiency:
    - prolonged ventilation (:> 2 weeks), e.g. severe chest trauma.
    - coma.
    - pulmonary diseases.
- Miscellaneous:
    - to decrease anatomic dead space.
    - to facilitate tracheobronchial lavage.
    - to assist in ventilator weaning.

Advantages of tracheostomy

- Improved patient comfort.
- Reduced incidence of accidental extubation.

- Easier airway suctioning and tracheobronchial toilet.

- Facilitates ventilation.

- Decreased sedative requirement.

- Increased airway efficiency (less dead space, lower resistance to air flow).

- Earlier ITU discharge.

- Facilitation of ventilator weaning.

Options

- Standard tracheostomy.

- Mini-tracheostomy (4 mm uncuffed tube, under local anaesthetic): for removal of secretions, inserted via cricothyroid membrane.

- Percutaneous: Seldinger technique, guidewire and dilators.

Surgical procedure

1 General anaesthetic, with an endotracheal tube.

2 Transverse collar incision.

3 Thyroid isthmus retracted upwards.

4 Pretracheal fascia incised.

5 Transverse incision between second and third tracheal rings.

Management

- Humidification of inspired air to prevent drying of the airway.

- Wound care and securing of tracheostomy tube.

- Regular wound swabs.

- Airway care.

- Frequent suctioning, by aseptic technique, to clear secretions.

- Nasogastric tube may be necessary if patient unable to swallow.

- Tube care:

  - outer tube replaced after 5 days (once track established).

  - inner tubes must be cleaned as necessary.

  - identical sized tube at bedside in case quick change necessary.

- Decannulation:
    - remove tube as soon as feasible.
    - tube spigoted for 24 h before removal.
    - stoma covered with dry occlusive dressing and allowed to heal spontaneously.

Complications

Complication rate varies from 6 to 51%:

- Immediate:
    - haemorrhage.
    - air embolus.
    - local structure damage:
        - carotid vessels.
        - recurrent laryngeal nerve.
        - oesophagus.
        - brachiocephalic vein.
    - apnoea.
    - misplacement.
- Continuing care:
    - wound infection.
    - tracheitis.
    - tracheal necrosis and mucosal damage.
    - tube blockage (prevent with humidified air).
    - tube displacement.
    - surgical emphysema.
    - pneumothorax and pneumomediastinum.
    - tracheal stenosis.
    - decannulation problems.
    - fistula:
        - tracheo-innominate artery fistula.
        - tracheo-oesophageal fistula.

Further reading

NJ Roland, McRae RDR, McCombe AW. *Key Topics in Otolaryngology*. Bios Scientific Publishers, Oxford 1995.

Cricothyroidotomy

- Technique of failure, when the patient cannot be intubated or ventilated.

- It is a temporising measure only: the patient still needs a definitive airway.

- Cricothyroid membrane (CTM) lies between the thyroid (Adam's apple) and cricoid cartilages, and is a relatively avascular structure.

Two techniques are described:

- Surgical cricothyroidotomy.

    1 longitudinal incision is made over the CTM, which is then incised with a scalpel blade under direct vision.

    2 small 4–5 mm tracheal tube is passed through the incision into the trachea, and connected to a breathing circuit for ventilation.

- Needle cricothyroidotomy:

    1 14 or 16 G venflon is attached to a 10 ml syringe and directed at 45° caudad.

    2 once the membrane is pierced, air is freely aspirated into the syringe, which indicates correct placement in the airway.

    3 cannula is passed over the needle and advanced distally into the airway.

    4 cannula is attached to a high-pressure (4 atm) wall oxygen supply.

    5 delivered for 1–2 s (watching the chest rise).

    6 5–6 s is needed for expiration via the patient's airway (the gauge of the cannula is too narrow to allow passive expiration).

Complications

- Subglottic stenosis.
- Tracheal stenosis.
- Intravascular placement.
- Pneumothorax/haemothorax.
- Infection.
- Oesophageal perforation.
- Pneumomediastinum.

INTERCOSTAL CHEST TUBE DRAINAGE

Indications

- Air/fluid in the pleural space leading to respiratory difficulty:
    - pneumothorax.
    - haemothorax.
    - empyema.
    - malignant effusion.
    - trauma.
- Prophylactic:
    - rib fractures.
    - mechanical ventilation (IPPV).
    - aeromedical evacuation.

Contraindications

Coagulopathy can lead to haemothorax formation.

Physiology

A chest drain is inserted to drain the pleural space and re-establish a negative intrapleural pressure.

Insertion

The authors advocate the insertion of the chest tube without a trocar (ATLS® technique):

1 Identify fifth intercostal space (nipple level) anterior to the mid-axillary line (higher in pregnant women).

2 Consent, sedation and local anaesthetic.

3 2–3 cm incision in the line of the rib.

4 Blunt dissection down through subcutaneous tissues over the top of the lower rib.

5 Puncture pleura with a clamp.

6 Finger sweep to clear adhesions, clots or debris from empyema.

7 Insert chest tube without trocar and connect to an underwater seal (acts as a one way valve).

8 Suture in place with a mattress suture.

9 Obtain a check CXR.

Continuing care

- Maintain the drain at a level below that of the patient.
- Clamp the drain when moving the patient.
- Blocked drains can lead to a tension pneumothorax.

Removal

Chest tubes should be removed when they no longer serve a purpose (namely no air or fluid is draining). The suitable time for removal is when:

- Bubbling has stopped for 24 h.
- There is no bubbling on coughing.
- CXR shows full expansion of the lung.

Complications

- Damage to thoracic or abdominal structures: this is almost universally by inserting the chest tube with a trocar.
- Infection (empyema).
- Neurovascular damage:
  - bleeding leading to haemothorax.
  - intercostal neuritis.
- Incorrect tube position:
  - extrapleural.
  - subdiaphragmatic.
- Tube complication:
  - blockage.
  - dislodgement.
  - disconnection.
- Persistent pneumothorax:
  - large primary leak.

- incomplete seal at skin.

- inadequate underwater seal.

- Subcutaneous emphysema: leak through parietal pleura but not through skin.

Cross-reference

Chapter 34, p. 322.   CSiG

Further reading

American College of Surgeons Committee on Trauma. *ATLS® Student Manual* (Chicago, American College of Surgeons, 1997).

BRONCHO-ALVEOLAR LAVAGE

This is a means of obtaining washings for microbiological analysis from the most distal parts of the respiratory tree. These procedures are performed on intubated, sedated patients. There are two ways to gain these samples:

- Under direct vision using a bronchoscope. This has the advantage of gaining samples from more distal aspects of the bronchial tree. The operator may also view the anatomy and take biopsies where necessary. It is, however, very invasive and requires considerable expertise.

- 'Blind' using a suction catheter and saline flush. This is a simpler and cheaper method, requiring minimal equipment and training. However, it is not usually possible to gain access to the distal parts of the bronchial tree.

DIAGNOSTIC PERITONEAL LAVAGE

Diagnostic peritoneal lavage (DPL) detects free intraperitoneal blood with 97% accuracy.

Definition

The washing out of the peritoneum for diagnostic purposes.

Indications

- Trauma:
    - altered consciousness: head injury; alcohol.

- altered sensation: spinal cord injury.

- injury to adjacent structures: lower rib fractures.

- equivocal surgical signs.

- stab wounds.

- Therapeutic uses of peritoneal lavage:

  - ascites drainage for respiratory compromise in malignancy.

  - alteration of core temperature ($\uparrow$ or $\downarrow$).

Contraindications

Contraindications to DPL are given in Table 6.1.

Table 6.1: Contraindications to DPL.

Absolute	Relative
Clinical indication for laparotomy Abdominal sepsis	Multiple previous abdominal operations Ileus Morbid obesity Advanced cirrhosis Pregnancy

Procedure

The landmark for incision is one-third of the way between umbilicus and symphysis pubis:

1 Drain stomach with nasogastric tube and bladder with urinary catheter.

2 Aseptic technique.

3 Via either open (preferred; obligatory in presence of pelvic fracture) or closed technique.

4 Local anaesthetic (lidocaine [lignocaine] + epinephrine [adrenaline]).

5 Incise skin and subcutaneous tissue in a longitudinal midline incision.

6 Grasp peritoneum with clamps and incise.

7 Advance dialysis catheter into pelvis.

8 Instil 1 litre warmed Hartmann's solution.

9 Gently agitate abdomen to ensure mixing.

10 Drain instilled fluid after 5–10 min.

11 Send drained fluid to laboratory for RBC and WBC counts.

Interpretation

The following indicate a POSITIVE test:

- > 10 ml frank blood.
- > 100 000 RBC ml^{-1}.
- > 500 WBC ml^{-1}.
- Bile/bowel contents drained from catheter.
- Gram +ve for bacteria.
- Peritoneal lavage fluid drained from catheter or chest tube.

Complications

- False-positive:
  - haemorrhage from surgical incision.
  - pelvic fracture.
- Perforation:
  - bladder.
  - bowel: leading to peritonitis.
- Missed retroperitoneal injury.
- Infection.

Further reading

American College of Surgeons Committee on Trauma *ATLS® Student Manual* (Chicago, American College of Surgeons, 1997).

INTRACRANIAL PRESSURE MONITORING

ICP monitoring is being increasingly used in the critical care setting. The principal use is after head injury. The lack of facilities to measure and monitor ICP should preclude a centre from managing severe head injury patients as they will be unable to maintain cerebral perfusion pressure accurately.

Indications

- Clinical signs obscured: drugs: sedatives, muscle relaxants.
- To assess when intervention is necessary:
  - severe head injury.
  - infection.
- Intensive care management of patients following traumatic brain injury.
- Measuring ICP enables calculation of cerebral perfusion pressure (CPP):

$$CPP = \text{mean arterial pressure} - ICP.$$

Contraindications

- Coagulopathy.
- Sepsis.

Insertion of ICP bolt

Measurement of ICP can be at four sites:

- Extradural.
- Subdural.
- Subarachnoid.
- Catheter in lateral ventricle.

Simultaneous measurements from various sites enable calculation of pressure gradients.

Bedside monitors enable visualisation of waveforms.

Intraventricular catheters allow treatment of raised ICP by drainage of CSF.

Most ICP bolts can be inserted under local anaesthetic at the bedside. The subdural bolt will be concentrated on, but the principles remain much the same:

1 A burr hole is drilled by standard technique.

2 A small hole is made in the dura mater.

3 The 'bolt' is inserted into the subdural space.

4 To enable monitoring, a transducer is connected to the bolt.

5 The bolt should be flushed infrequently with 0.1 ml N saline (0.9% NaCl).

Complications

- Infection.
- Bleeding → intracranial collection/haematoma.
- Screw end obstruction → loss of reliable ICP measurement.

Cross-reference

Chapter 2, p. 39.   CSiG

Matta BF, Menon DK. Monitoring the brain after severe head   SURGERY
injury. *Surgery* 1998; 16: 16–19.

Further reading

Andrews PJD, Souter MJ. *Recent Advances in the Management of Traumatic Brain Injury: Current Practice in Critical Illness* (London: Chapman & Hall, 1996).
Soni N. *Practical Procedures in Anaesthesia and Intensive Care* (Oxford: Butterworth-Heinemann, 1989).

PERICARDIAL ASPIRATION

Indications

- Diagnostic: suspected pericardial effusion.
- Therapeutic: cardiac tamponade.

Contraindications

There are no contraindications to alleviating life-threatening cardiac tamponade.

Technique

The procedure should usually be performed under echocardiographic guidance:

1 Attach ECG monitoring, position patient 35–45° head up.

2 Local anaesthetic as appropriate.

3 Puncture skin 2 cm below the angle between xiphisternum and seventh costal cartilage.

4 Advance long needle at 45° aiming for the left shoulder.

5 Slowly advance drawing back on the syringe.

6 Observe monitor for ectopics or ST segment changes.

7 Aspirate effusion to dryness (aspiration of a 20 ml effusion can result in a dramatic improvement in cardiac output)

Monitoring

- Heart rate and ECG trace for procedure.

- Blood pressure every 15 min for 2 h after the procedure.

Complications

- Puncture of adjacent structures:

  - lung: pneumothorax.

  - oesophagus: mediastinitis (see Chapter 4).

  - peritoneum: peritonitis.

- Dramatic decrease in heart rate (vagal stimulation): stop aspiration: arrhythmias leading to VF: stop aspiration.

- Dry aspiration: ? fluid too viscous.

- Haemorrhage: laceration of ventricles, coronary vessels, or great vessels necessitating thoracotomy.

A pericardial window under general anaesthetic or a formal thoracotomy and pericardiotomy are both more effective than needle pericardiocentesis.

Further reading

ATLS® Student Manual (American College of Surgeons, 1997).

INTRA-ABDOMINAL PRESSURE (IAP) MONITORING

IAP is an important measure of underlying abdominal problems and an indicator of a patient's physiological status. Monitoring of IAP in the critically ill is gaining favour. Slight increases in IAP have been shown to have deleterious effects on organ function.

Uses

- Indicator of abdominal compartment syndrome (ACS).

- Guide to performing a second-look laparotomy.

- Guide to leaving the abdomen open after laparotomy.

Normal IAP

Subatmospheric (< 0 mmHg).

Technique

The Cheatham and Safesak modification of Kron's technique is simple and safe:

1 Connect Luer lock syringe and transducer via a cannula in the culture aspiration port to an intravesical Foley catheter.

2 Prime with normal saline and zero at the level of the symphysis pubis.

3 Clamp catheter distal to culture aspiration port.

4 Instil 50 ml normal saline into the bladder.

5 Allow to equilibrate.

6 Measure IAP at end-expiration.

7 Unclamp catheter.

Clinical importance of IAP

- IAP > 10 mmHg has been demonstrated to be instrumental in organ dysfunction. Intra-abdominal hypertension (IAH; > 25 mmHg) is deleterious to both intra- and extra-abdominal organs. IAH is an independent risk factor for ITU mortality rate and has been demonstrated in 30% of a surgical ITU population.

- Raised IAP affects chest wall mechanics and decompression has beneficial effects on respiratory mechanics and oxygenation.

Complications

- Urinary tract infection.
- Sepsis.

Further reading

Malbrain MLNG. Abdominal pressure in the critically ill: measurement and clinical relevance. *Intensive Care Medicine* 1999; 25: 1453–8.

Cross-reference

Schein M. The stuffed turkey syndrome. *Surgery* 1999; 17: i–ii.   SURGERY

INDEX